DR DAWN HARPER

LIVE WELL TO 101

QUICK AND EASY DAILY TIPS FOR A LONG AND HEALTHY LIFE

Copyright © 2018 Dawn Harper

The right of Dawn Harper to be identified as the Author of the Work has been asserted by her in accordance with the Copyright, Designs and Patents Act 1988.

First published in Great Britain in 2018 by HEADLINE HOME an imprint of HEADLINE PUBLISHING GROUP

First published in paperback in 2019

1

Cataloguing in Publication Data is available from the British Library

Paperback ISBN 978 1 4722 4865 7

Typeset in Gill Sans Std by Palimpsest Book Production Ltd, Falkirk, Stirlingshire

Printed and bound by Clays Ltd, Elcograf S.p.A

MIX
Paper from
responsible sources
FSC® C104740

Headline's policy is to use papers that are natural, renewable and recyclable products and made from wood grown in sustainable forests. The logging and manufacturing processes are expected to conform to the environmental regulations of the country of origin.

HEADLINE PUBLISHING GROUP
An Hachette UK Company
Carmelite House
50 Victoria Embankment
London EC4Y 0DZ

www.headline.co.uk
www.hachette.co.uk

Thanks to Victor van Amerongen
for all his invaluable research,
without which this book would
still be just a twinkle in my eye.

CONTENTS

INTRODUCTION

We are living longer. A girl born in the UK today can expect to live beyond her 83rd birthday, and a boy halfway into his 80th year. But living long doesn't necessarily mean living *well*. I have met far too many elderly people who have little or no quality of life, and many people who fear old age because they've watched their loved ones deteriorate physically and mentally in later life.

I really believe it doesn't have to be that way.

In this book I am going to show you how you can invest now for your later years to improve your chances of enjoying them to the full. There are two lovely quotations – I don't know where they originated, but I'd like to remind you of them now. The first is: 'I don't want to arrive at the pearly gates wearing incontinence pads and dribbling, in a wheelchair. I want to screech in wearing purple, a glass of champagne in hand, saying "Thank you for the ride!"'

We may want to receive a card from the Queen on our 100th birthday – but we would also want to be aware of the significance of the card, and remember who the Queen is. I also doubt many of us want to work towards a healthy old age but make our younger years a misery in the process. And this is where the second quote comes in: 'Giving up everything you enjoy doesn't actually make you live longer; it just feels like you do!'

That is precisely why I wanted to write this book. There is nothing in here that will recommend a hideously restrictive diet or living your life as though you are training for a marathon or about to climb Mount Everest. In fact, this book does the exact opposite. It shows you how small, achievable and sustainable changes really can alter your future.

I have always said that there is no such thing as an unhealthy food, but there are plenty of unhealthy diets – and in this book I show you exactly what I mean. In my over 21 years in general practice, I have gained hundreds of simple tips for living longer, and living better, all of which can make a significant difference if you incorporate them into your life. I want to share these tips with you now. I think you will be pleasantly surprised by how easy some are to achieve.

Before I start, let me show you what I mean by living well into old age. Let me introduce you to a patient of mine. Ethel married her childhood sweetheart, an army man a few years her junior. When I first met them they were celebrating 60 years of what was clearly a very happy marriage. Her modest flat is filled with pictures of him in uniform. Her late husband was one of my first patients when I joined my practice. He was a very dignified gentleman, and when I met him he was in the last stages of his battle with cancer. Sadly, he came to the end of his journey but, fifteen years on, Ethel is still going strong.

Aged 100, she walks the half-mile to surgery to see me. She lives in a warden-controlled apartment adjoining a nursing home. She has no help, does her own food shopping, cooks her own meals and cleans her own home – which, by the way, is always immaculate on the odd occasion she requests a home visit. She regularly plays the rather magnificent grand piano that has pride of place in her living room, and she sings. Ethel was an amateur opera singer in her youth and despite her age still holds a note beautifully.

She has one son, who lives in Australia. With no family nearby, Christmas can be a difficult time for her, and as I have got to know her I always ask her about her plans for Christmas. Last year she replied simply, 'I have agreed to sing for the old folk next door.' I smiled inside – partly because I knew what a treat the 'old folk' were in for, but mainly because some of those 'old folk' would be twenty years her junior! Yet again I was reminded of the sometimes cavernous difference between chronological and biological age.

So what has enabled Ethel to live an active life into her second century? Is it down to luck and good genes, or can we really alter our life expectancy by what we eat, where we live, what we earn, or how we look at life?

I believe we can. I can't guarantee that by following the advice in this book you will live until you're 101, but I *know* that by making some changes today you should be able to live a happier, more fulfilled life tomorrow and beyond.

Think of it as a pension policy. The earlier you start paying in, the more you stand to gain. If you start paying into a pension scheme in your twenties, your pension pot will be bigger by the time you decide to retire, allowing you a much better standard of living. If you wait until middle age before you start thinking about pensions, you will have less to enjoy – and if you have no policy and leave everything to luck, you could find yourself in trouble.

It's the same with health. The earlier you start to invest in your own longevity, the more likely you are not just to live longer but to live your later years in good health and enjoying a better quality of life.

As an NHS GP, I am often asked to visit patients in nursing homes. I can think of two homes less than a mile apart. Whenever I visit one, I can't help feeling overwhelming sadness. It is as if time has stopped and the residents are simply 'waiting for God'. Just up the hill is the other home, where there are almost as many pets as there are residents – dogs, cats, rabbits and even a tortoise! There are regular exercise classes: granted, some residents enjoy these from a chair, but they are joyous occasions – as are the music evenings, the bingo and the regular outings. The residents in the second home seem so much more fulfilled, and many are still enjoying life well into their nineties.

You can either accept your decline – or celebrate your later years. The second nursing home I mentioned above feels like a club – one that I would like for myself, or for members of my family, when the time comes.

We know that life expectancy has risen for generations, but I'm not as interested in how long we live, as in how well we live.

In my GP practice we have a Christmas party in the village hall for the over-75s. Each year we invite all our patients aged over 75 to the party and they come along to enjoy sandwiches, cakes, a cup of tea and a tot of sherry. It's usually something of a riot, but we have had to have serious discussions in the practice about whether we need to increase the entry age to 85, since more and more people are living beyond 75 and we could get to the stage where we just can't accommodate all of those who are eligible.

There is another side to this, though. Sadly, not all our over-75s can attend the party. Some are too incapacitated to join us. They may be living a long time, but the quality of those extra years is poor. I doubt any of us want to live years – or, heaven forbid, decades – in chronic pain or without the mental capacity to enjoy that longevity. I want to be able to go dancing in the village hall at Christmas and I want the same for my friends, my family and for you. So, whether you are picking this book up for yourself, for your parents, or even for your children, I want to show you how you can increase your chances of living into a vibrant old age.

In this book, I will also introduce you to some wonderful centenarians for whom age really is just a number, and let them tell you what they think is the secret to their thriving old age. I will take you step by step through all the things that can influence how well we live in our later decades, and give you my top tips on how to achieve this for yourself and for your family.

Along the way I will try to answer these questions:

- Is your lifespan simply predetermined by your genes?
- Can a healthy lifestyle dramatically improve your chances of reaching a very old age?
- Is longevity affected by where you live, the car you drive, your choice of pet, or your level of sexual activity?
- Can you pay your way to living longer with private healthcare or expensive medical scans?

I want to assess the major factors that determine how long we live and give some practical advice on the measures we can all take to beat the odds and live significantly longer.

However, this isn't just about long life – it's about having a great life and drawing on the wisdom of those who are living the latter stages of their life with joy, health and happiness.

I will also be reporting on the latest scientific research into ways that people all over the world are achieving not just a longer life, but a better quality of life, as they reach their second century. I want to show how you can plan ahead – not just for longevity, but for a happy, healthy and active long life.

In short, I will tell you how to live well – not just today and tomorrow and next year, but all the way to 101!

Did you know the following facts?

- Women are more likely to die in the week after their birthday than at any other time of the year.
- In the UK, the richest 5% of men live an average of 34.2 years longer than the poorest 5%.
- Smoking still accounts for over 96,000 deaths in the UK every year.
- People who are slightly overweight live longer than people who are the ideal weight.
- The highest incidence of fatal heart attacks occurs on Christmas Day.

- Type 2 diabetes reduces your life expectancy by an average of ten years.
- The murder rate in Scotland is almost double that in England and Wales.
- Motorcyclists are 38 times more likely to die in a UK road accident than car drivers.

Here's a quick guide to what you'll find in each chapter of this book.

Chapter 1: Meet the centenarians

I start by meeting some remarkable people who have already lived to 100 or more – people who have also managed to maintain an active and healthy lifestyle along the way. I also take a look at the latest research into ageing. Is it possible that future generations could live for hundreds of years?

Chapter 2: The luck of the dice?

Is your lifespan just a matter of having good or bad genes? Although genetic factors play a significant role, lifestyle factors are far more important in setting you on the path to a long life and long-term good health.

Chapter 3: Cigarettes and alcohol

Let's start by addressing the obvious risk factors. Just how bad are your bad habits in the long term? How can you break free from dependence on smoking, drinking or drugs? And, if you do achieve a better lifestyle, can you undo the harm you've already done?

Chapter 4: Diabetes – a twenty-first-century epidemic

Type 2 diabetes is becoming an epidemic in the developed world. It is claiming lives prematurely and leaving many more people with a poor quality of life as a result of complications of the disease. In this chapter I will tell you how to reduce your risk of developing the disease.

Chapter 5: Good diets, bad diets

In this chapter I will show you exactly what we mean by a healthy, well balanced diet, what a portion really should look like, and how to look out for hidden fat, sugar and salt in the food we eat.

Chapter 6: Let's get physical

Around 44% of adults in the UK do little or no regular exercise. This chapter discusses the various types of exercise available, whether you're a gym bunny or a hiker. What type of exercise is most effective? This chapter shows you that even modest changes to your daily routine can make a big difference to your health.

Chapter 7: A healthy heart

Coronary heart disease is the leading cause of death in the UK and worldwide. How important are genetic factors? What are the risk factors associated with raised cholesterol, high blood pressure, angina, or an abnormal heart rhythm? And how can you change or adapt your lifestyle to prevent – or even reverse – heart disease? With an ageing population, dementia is on the rise. Do we just accept this as part of the ageing process, or can we reduce our risk factors and help to prevent dementia?

Chapter 8: The battle against cancer

Although the group of diseases collectively known as 'cancer' accounts for about 15% of all deaths, survival rates for many cancers are improving dramatically year by year. To what extent are the different cancers caused by inherited genetics or environmental factors? And how can you modify your lifestyle to reduce your risk?

Chapter 9: Your best shot

There has been a lot of bad press around vaccination in the UK, but vaccination is probably one of the greatest medical developments in modern-day Britain. This chapter explains the vaccination schedule in the UK, and describes the diseases the vaccines protect against.

Chapter 10: Mind over matter

Since optimists seem to live longer than pessimists, how does your attitude affect your long-term health? Find out how the 'will to live' acts as both a conscious and an unconscious mechanism to help people overcome serious injury or disease. Also, discover how your relationships, friendships and sex life can play an important part in maintaining your health.

Chapter 11: A place to grow old

This chapter looks at Acciaroli in Italy, which is famous for the longevity of its residents. It also covers the risk factors that can (perhaps surprisingly) affect your health – where you live, the countries you visit, your hobbies and interests, the pets you keep, and the type of job you do.

Chapter 12: Money matters

There is a huge gap in life expectancy between the richest and poorest people in the UK. Why is this, and is there anything you can do about it? Is the answer to have constant medical supervision (as members of the Royal Family do)? How effective are CT and MRI scans at picking up early signs of life-threatening diseases? Does having access to private medicine give you a huge advantage?

Chapter 13: The elixir of life

This chapter assesses all the risk factors covered in this book and pulls together my top tips on how to achieve a long, healthy life.

Chapter 14: And finally . . .

This chapter summarises some slightly less scientific theories about the factors that affect our longevity.

CHAPTER 1

MEET THE CENTENARIANS

Hadlow Castle was an imposing eighteenth-century country house built in an ornate Gothic style a few miles south-east of London in rural Kent. Although the main building was largely demolished in 1951, the octagonal Hadlow Tower survives along with a variety of stables and the servants' quarters. Even so, local people still refer to the remaining buildings as Hadlow Castle.

Jimmy Thirsk has lived there since 1954. Every Monday he leaves his home and takes the bus into Tonbridge, about four miles away, to visit the supermarket and stock up on supplies of his favourite food – fish.

'I eat a lot of fish,' he tells me. 'For lunch I have tinned sardines on toast. For dinner I fry up plaice, haddock or cod. I even eat those tiny bits of raw herring – I love them.'

Jimmy has just celebrated his 102nd birthday. I recently visited him one sunny afternoon, and enjoyed a cup of tea in his book-lined study. This reflects his lengthy career as a librarian: 'Libraries are tranquil places and I wouldn't have been happy in any job that wasn't concerned with books.'

It's one thing to live to an advanced age. But I've rarely met anyone who seems to be in such good health, or with such a relaxed attitude to life and death. 'You had the chance of living,' he says, 'and you've lived a long life, so why worry about going?'

He certainly comes from a family that defies the odds. 'My grandfather was 81; he died in 1905. And my great-grandfather Thirsk was 86 when he died in 1880. My mother had seven sisters and two brothers, and one lived to be 101 and four of them lived to be in their nineties. So I think there are good genes on all sides.' His sister also died at the age of 101.

Jimmy shows no signs of slowing down. His first book (a memoir of his time at Bletchley Park during World War II) was published when he was 94. He is now working on an autobiography. He still travels to London by train, takes holidays, and keeps in touch with his friends by email.

So maybe it's the genes, the fishy diet or, as he tells me, 'a combination of luck and the National Health Service'. Or perhaps Jimmy's real secret is his calm temperament, because in his 102 years he has only lost his temper once. ' I was waiting for a bus and leaning against a lamp post for support. And an old man came by and said "You shouldn't lean on that thing." And I thought "you so-and-so" and told him in a few harsh words what I thought about him. And that's the only time I can remember losing my temper.'

Slightly younger is 100-year-old Jean Dawson from Cottingley, West Yorkshire. Her passion is Iyengar yoga.

Jean started going to yoga classes when she was 67, and the benefits are plain to see. 'It has really changed my life and has helped cure aches and pains,' she says. Going to regular classes has also done wonders for her social life. 'I have met many kind people through yoga and made some good friends. I don't know how I would be today if I hadn't taken up Iyengar yoga. It has given me good posture, balance, concentration, flexibility and stamina.'

Her early life gives no clues to the long, healthy life she would lead. Jean Dawson was born in London in 1916, but was adopted after her father died. She says that she didn't do any sports or exercise when she was young, but now the grandmother of five and great-grandmother of two, who served in the Land Army during World War II, intends to go on bending and twisting her body for as long as she can. 'I really enjoy the company,' she says, 'so I think I can continue for a little longer.'

According to her yoga teacher, Christine Tyson (who is a mere 66), Jean is a real inspiration to the younger members of the group: 'Jean is a role model in class – if Jean can do it, so can the class.'

MANY HAPPY RETURNS

Jimmy Thirsk and Jean Dawson seem to have defied the odds – not just by living to a very old age, but also by remaining sufficiently well to go on enjoying an active lifestyle. But stories like these are much more common than they used to be because life expectancy continues to rise at a dramatic rate.

In any high-street newsagent you can find a selection of birthday cards for 100-year-olds. They show pictures of cakes, candles, flowers and balloons, and they carry cheerful messages – 'Looking Totally Fabulous at 100', 'Happy 100th, You Made It!' and 'Keep calm, you're only 100!' Retail shops are not in the business of giving shelf space to products that don't sell, so there is clearly a demand for them.

Queen Elizabeth II may be regretting the tradition of sending a congratulatory message to anyone in the UK who's celebrating their 100th birthday. This custom was started in 1917 by King George V. Until fairly recently, the messages were sent as telegrams by the Royal Mail's Inland Telegram Service.

The design of the telegrams changed over the years, but the message itself stayed much the same: 'I am so pleased to know that you are celebrating your 100th birthday. I send my congratulations and best wishes to you on such a special occasion.' The message now takes the form of a laser-printed card bearing a photo of the monarch. Whereas there were originally only a handful of centenarians to congratulate every year, the Anniversaries Office at Buckingham Palace now sends out around 8,000 100th birthday cards annually – an increase of 350% in just 30 years. So, in statistical terms, I could reasonably claim that '100 is the new 80'.

WE'RE ALL LIVING LONGER

According to the most recent government figures, the average life expectancy in England and Wales for a baby born this year is 83.2 years for a girl and 79.5 years for a boy. These figures are actually for life expectancy at birth – the average age that a baby born in this country at this time can expect to live. (Table 13.1 gives information on life expectancy in the UK.)

We know that in prehistoric times, life expectancy was 20–30 years. In Sweden in the 1750s it was 36 years, and in 1900 the average life expectancy in the USA was 48.

These figures may paint a slightly misleading picture because they suggest that there were no old people at all. Until fairly recently, infant mortality was a major factor in skewing life expectancy figures. Infant Mortality Rate (IMR) is usually defined as the death of a child before their first birthday. In seventeenth-century Europe, the IMR was between 20% and 40%. It varied dramatically from year to year as countries were affected by epidemics, famines and wars.

Even in the nineteenth century, the chances of a child surviving that critical first year were not great. In the summer of 1876 the *New York Times* reported that in Manhattan over 100 infants were dying every day because of a particularly virulent outbreak of gastroenteritis. In the Victorian era, people planned to have large families in the expectation that some of their children (about one in every three in urban areas) would die before reaching adulthood.

In the UK today, the IMR is – thankfully – less than 0.5%, and falling. That's one reason why life expectancies all over the world are continuing to increase so dramatically.

According to the World Health Organization (WHO), in 1955 the worldwide average life expectancy was just 48 years. By 1995 it was 65 years, and by 2025 it is expected to reach 73 years.

However, there are huge variations from one part of the world to another. Table 1.1 shows the ten countries with the highest life expectancies.

Table 1.1: The ten countries with the highest life expectancies. Reproduced with permission of the World Health Organization. Taken from **www.who.int/gho/publications/world_health_statistics/2016/Annex_B/en/** (World Health Statistics 2016: Monitoring health for the SDGs. Annex B: tables of health statistics by country, WHO region and globally).

Country	Overall rank	Overall life expectancy	Female rank	Female life expectancy	Male rank	Male life expectancy
Japan	1	84	1	87	6	80
Spain	2	83	2	86	6	80
Andorra	2	83	2	86	16	79
Singapore	2	83	4	85	2	81
Switzerland	2	83	4	85	2	81
Australia	2	83	4	85	6	80
Italy	2	83	4	85	6	80
San Marino	2	83	11	84	1	83
France	9	82	4	85	16	79
Monaco	9	82	4	85	16	79

Again according to the WHO, Table 1.2 shows the countries with the lowest life expectancies.

Interestingly, women live an average of 3.9 years longer than men. But this statistical pattern, which is widely regarded as the norm, is a relatively recent phenomenon. According to the University of Southern California, the trend began around 1870, when deaths from infectious diseases became less common and more deaths were linked to cancer and cardiovascular diseases, which affect men more than women. But now the trend is going in the other direction.

Men's life expectancies are catching up. And, in some places, men consistently outlive women by a wide margin. In the relatively affluent neighbourhood of Bewbush and Broadfield in West Sussex, England, men can expect to live to 96, while women reach an average age of only 83.

So everyone everywhere is living longer, and men are (on average) catching up with women. And that's why there are so many more centenarians.

Table 1.2: The ten countries with the lowest life expectancies. Reproduced with permission of the World Health Organization. Taken from **www.who.int/gho/publications/world_health_statistics/2016/Annex_B/en/** (World Health Statistics 2016: Monitoring health for the SDGs. Annex B: tables of health statistics by country, WHO region and globally).

Country	Overall rank	Overall life expectancy	Female rank	Female life expectancy	Male rank	Male life expectancy
Guinea-Bissau	184	54	184	55	184	53
Mozambique	184	54	184	55	184	53
Côte d'Ivoire	187	53	187	54	188	52
Swaziland	187	53	189	53	184	53
Democratic Republic of the Congo	189	52	187	54	189	51
Chad	189	52	189	53	189	51
Angola	189	52	189	53	191	50
Central African Republic	192	51	192	52	191	50
Lesotho	193	50	192	52	193	48
Sierra Leone	194	46	194	46	194	46

WHO IS THE OLDEST PERSON IN THE WORLD?

According to the United Nations, there are around 400,000 centenarians alive in the world today. The figure is inexact because data from many countries is sketchy or unreliable – and 100 years ago, when these people were being born, not all countries kept accurate birth records.

We do know with more accuracy that the USA has the greatest number of proven centenarians – 53,364, according to the most recent census in 2010. Japan has the second highest, with 51,376. (Note that Japan's population is only around 40% that of the USA!)

However, if you do make it to 100, you shouldn't expect to live a great deal beyond that. In fact, only 1 in 1,000 centenarians lives to become 110 – a so-called 'supercentenarian'.

Although worldwide there are thought to be around 500 supercentenarians, only 50 such claims can be fully verified. Of these, 49 are women.

If you make it to the age of 114 years and 28 days, you can boast that you have been alive for one million hours. And if you make it to 123, you will officially be the oldest person who ever lived, beating Jeanne Calment from Arles in France, who died in 1997 at the age of 122. What an amazing life she had! Born on 21 February 1875, she was the daughter of parents who lived for a long time (Nicolas, 1837–1931 and Marguerite, 1838–1924). Jeanne lived to see the invention of cars, planes and television. The Eiffel Tower – at that time the world's tallest building – opened when she was 14, and she lived through both world wars.

Jeanne Calment also met Vincent van Gogh when she was thirteen. The great Dutch artist came into her father's shop in Arles to buy some coloured pencils – but she didn't take to him, complaining that he was scruffy and smelled of alcohol. She put her long life down to 'olive oil, port and chocolate'. However, she also smoked, although she finally gave up in 1995, two years before her death.

Of course, whenever a person lives to a great age they become something of a celebrity, and are asked what their secret is. Here's what some centenarians have had to say:

Filomena Taipe Mendoza (117, Peru): 'A natural diet of potatoes, goat's milk, goat cheese and beans.'

Misao Okawa (117, Japan): 'Be nice to other people, the way you want them to be nice to you.'

Besse Cooper (116, USA): 'Don't eat junk food. Treat everyone the way you want to be treated.'

Emma Morano (116, Italy): 'Eat three eggs a day, drink a glass of homemade brandy, and think positively about the future.'

Christian Mortensen (115, USA): 'Friends, a good cigar, drinking lots of good water, no alcohol and lots of singing.'

Laila Denmark (114, USA): 'Eat right and do what you love. Whatever you love to do is play; doing what you don't like to do is work.'

Bonita Zigrang (110, USA): 'Have a good appetite, lots of friends, and keep busy.'

I'm not claiming this gives us any scientific information about the reasons for extreme longevity. These supercentenarians are at the statistical extreme, and it would be almost impossible to draw any meaningful conclusions from these subjective assessments. However, when you consider data collected about ageing from much larger groups, observed over long periods of time, you begin to be able to draw some robust conclusions about why some people live for such a long time.

THE STUDY OF AGEING

People have always been fascinated by the disparities in human longevity. As long ago as the tenth century, Arabic physician Ahmed Ibn Al-Jazzar (c.895–c.979) wrote about his studies of the elderly, giving advice on sleep disorders, forgetfulness and how to improve memory.

The term 'gerontology' as the study of ageing was coined in 1903 by Elie Metchnikoff, a Russian zoologist. It gained further respectability as a science when the Gerontological Society of America was founded in 1945. Gerontology was originally about studying the effects of ageing, both on the individual and on society, but from the 1960s onwards scientists began to investigate 'biogerontology'. This is the study of the ageing process itself – and what can be done to change it.

Cynthia Kenyon (b. 1954), a biogerontologist at the University of California, has shown that the lifespans of various types of worm and fruit fly can be dramatically extended by modifying their diet. Although this research has not yet been directly tested on humans, Ms Kenyon does at least practise what she preaches. She has adopted a low-carbohydrate diet like the Atkins diet, and she's very pleased with her results: 'I have a fabulous blood profile. My triglyceride level is only 30, and anything below 200 is good,' she said. 'Plus I feel better. Plus I'm thin. I weigh what I weighed when I was in college. I feel great – you feel like you're a kid again. It's amazing.'

Cynthia Kenyon also experimented with the 5:2 diet (in which you fast for two days of the week), but says she gave it up because she couldn't stand the constant hunger.

Biogerontologists believe that if we could understand what makes human beings age, we could intervene in the process to make people live longer. But there is disagreement about how effective this is likely to be. Professor Leonard Hayflick, author of *How and Why We Age*, believes that worldwide life expectancies will continue to rise, but that they will peak at around 92 years of age.[2] Another American scientist, James Vaupel, believes that the human lifespan is not fixed, and that children born today in Western countries can reasonably expect to live to an average of over 100.[3]

Aubrey de Grey, a molecular biologist from the University of Cambridge, goes much further. 'We have a 50/50 chance of developing technology within about 25 to 30 years from now that will . . . allow us to stop people from dying at any age.'[4] He believes life expectancies of 1,000 years are within scientific reach.

The easiest way to live to 101 (or substantially more) would be for science to discover what causes ageing, and then stop or reverse it. There are two theories for why we age:

- **The damage concept** – Over a period of many years our cells suffer genetic damage, including mutations to the DNA sequence. Our bodies are literally degraded by wear and tear, and eventually fail.
- **Programmed ageing** – This is based on the belief that an 'ageing clock' is built into the operation of the body's nervous or endocrine system. In other words, from the moment we are born we are pre-programmed to fail at some stage.

Today, the causes of ageing are still largely unknown, but I believe there is a consensus among scientists that the process doesn't have to be inevitable, and that we may well reach a point when we can use science to change our destinies. In other species, there is evidence that immortality is achievable. Small freshwater animals called hydra have the ability to regenerate themselves – they appear not to age or to die of old age. Now scientists from all over the world are competing to hack the code and discover what regulates our lifespan. Launched in 2014, the Palo Alto Longevity Prize will award $1,000,000 to the individual or team that succeeds in ending ageing.

The scientific way to extend our lives would probably be based on stem cell therapy and molecular regeneration. These techniques would enable doctors and scientists to identify, repair or even replace failing organs. (A vintage car can be kept on the road almost indefinitely if various engine parts are replaced. In the end the car may have been completely renewed, with none of the original parts remaining.)

According to one school of thought – the so-called 'longevity escape velocity' theory – we may already be at the point of being able to use this new science to extend our lives indefinitely. We would identify a group of healthy people who are aged 40–50, and apply existing knowledge to ensure they live for another 30 years. By then, the science of ageing will have improved so much that they will be able to benefit from new techniques that will rejuvenate them for a further 30 years. As therapies improve, they will again be able to escape the effects of ageing. In other words, the science could advance so fast that it stays ahead of our actual life cycle and we go on to live forever – or at least until we are killed by some non-medical occurrence such as a car crash or a lightning strike. (Statistically, if every disease were eliminated, the average person would live to be around 700 years old.)

I know that many people worry about the social consequences of greatly extended lifespans, but this view is not shared by Aubrey de Grey. 'The mistake people always make is that they think I'm saying we would live much longer in a context where nothing else changes,' he says. 'For example, people always panic about paying pensions to people that live longer. But why would you need a pension if you're healthy? Even the very concept of work won't exist in the same way, because we'll probably have more and more automation. Look, we have at least one hundred years before we'll have any 200-year-old people.'[5]

COLD COMFORT

If you're passing through Scottsdale, Arizona, any time soon you might like to reserve your place on a free guided tour of the Alcor Life Extension Foundation. Its website says that your tour will include 'viewing of our operating room, cooldown bay, and Patient Care Bay', as well as 'discussion of the history of Alcor, the cryopreservation process, and answers to your questions'. The tour lasts an hour, and you can pick up an application form if you like what you see.

Alcor is the world's largest cryopreservation facility – the process of freezing the human body after death in the expectation that people can be brought back to life at some future date when science makes that possible.

Max More, Alcor's President and CEO, certainly believes in his own product – he has signed up for a place in the deep freeze. 'I figure the future is a pretty decent place to be, so I want to be there,' he says. 'I want to keep living and enjoying and producing.'[6]

It seems that there are hundreds of people all over the world who like the idea of immortality, but who have given up on waiting for twenty-first-century science to give them that chance. Alcor is more than happy to supply potential applicants with 'fascinating details of the cryopreservation process'. As soon as you're declared legally dead, Alcor's team transfers your body to an ice bed and then uses a heart-lung resuscitator to get the blood flowing through your body again. They then administer sixteen different medications designed to protect your cells from deteriorating after death. This is all completely legal because you are (at this stage at least) dead.

The next step involves draining as much blood and other fluids as possible from your body, and replacing them with a type of antifreeze solution that won't form potentially damaging ice crystals when frozen.

Once your body is full of antifreeze, Alcor gradually cools you down over a two-week period until you eventually reach −196°C.

You will then be placed upside down in one of Alcor's frozen flasks, called dewars.

There you will remain in suspended animation, waiting to be revived at some point in the future. Max More reckons that will probably be in 50 to 100 years. 'But it's really impossible to say. We don't even know what repair technology would be used.[7]

The prospect of waking up in a future world where all your friends and family have long since died is my idea of a nightmare – but around 1,000 people have signed up so far to pay Alcor $200,000 to be cryopreserved. If you can't afford this, you can pay a discounted rate of $80,000 and just preserve your brain.

A LONG AND HEALTHY LIFE

We could wait for science to hand us the gift of immortality, either in the next few years or at some point in the distant future, but the factors that will determine the lifespan and well-being of most people are rather more mundane, but also more practical.

Our perceptions about ageing change as we age. This is largely linked to an individual's state of health. If people are well, they tend to be much more positive about getting older.[8] Fortunately, it seems that most people are quite relaxed about the idea of ageing, whatever age they are. According to a BBC survey,[9] most people aged 16–24 think that old age begins at 60. But when people aged 65 were asked the same question, they said old age began at 80. In scientific terms, 'old age' is often defined as the age when you have ten years of life expectancy left, so in the UK that would be around 70–75 years.

The idea of living to an old age is not universally appealing. In 2013 a survey by the USA's Pew Research Center[10] asked people if they would like to live until they were 120. Over half (56%) of adults said no, although roughly two-thirds (68%) thought that most other people would answer yes. When you look more deeply into the figures, it becomes clear that most people who dislike the idea of living to an old age do so because they associate it with ill health, becoming weak and needy, and being unable to carry out simple everyday tasks.

I think Shakespeare summed it up pretty well in *As You Like It.* He said old age: 'Is second childishness and mere oblivion/Sans teeth, sans eyes, sans taste, sans everything'.

This view is not shared by Jimmy Thirsk and Jean Dawson, who we met at the start of this chapter. They are clearly enjoying life as they enter their eleventh decade, so the simple achievement of reaching a certain age is only part of the story. We need to find ways to make sure we stay healthy and fit so that we have a good quality of life in our old age.

That's why life expectancy (LE) statistics are now often accompanied by measurements of healthy life expectancy (HLE) – the estimate of how many years an individual or a population might expect to live while also enjoying either 'good' or 'very good' health. According to the most recent figures from the Office for National Statistics, the HLE figure in England is 63.4 years for males and 64.1 years for females. Again, there are wide variations between areas. In the London borough of Tower Hamlets, the HLE for men is only 52.5 years, while for females living in Wokingham it is 71.0 years.

In most parts of the UK, the HLE figure is lower than the state pension age, which means (somewhat depressingly) that by the time you retire you're very likely to be in poor health. Also, the gap between the LE and HLE figures has grown in recent years. In the past 20 years, life expectancy has risen by 4.6%, but healthy life expectancy has only risen by 3.0%. In other words, although people are living longer, those extra years are often blighted by physical or mental impairment.

There is also a marked difference between the experiences of men and women: in this case British men do better, with an average of 80% of their lives spent enjoying good health, compared to 77% for women.

This simply underlines the point that striving to reach a great age is all very well, but it has to be accompanied by a sufficiently good quality of life to make it desirable.

LATE BLOOMERS

In the BBC survey mentioned above, a group of 250 adults of all ages was asked to say at what age they would like to retire. More than two-thirds chose 60 or below, which is of course younger than the official retirement age. In the same group, a large majority of adults aged over 35 said they were looking forward to retirement. When the BBC asked people who were already retired whether they were enjoying it, the unanimous response was 'it's great'.

Chapter 10 looks in more detail at the relationship between work and longevity. However, there is evidence that – despite what the above BBC survey found – retirement can actually be detrimental to long-term good health. Conversely, many people who go on working into their advancing years seem to enjoy better health, because they are keeping mentally and physically active.

I only have to switch on the TV or radio to see examples of people who have continued to work very effectively well past the normal retirement age. Mary Berry is now over 80, but she remains a popular presenter of BBC cookery programmes. At the age of 90, David Attenborough started work as narrator and presenter on a sequel to *The Blue Planet*, a nature documentary series he made in 2006 (when he was just 79). And Nicholas Parsons is still hosting *Just a Minute* on Radio 4 as he heads towards his 94th birthday.

These are people who have had a successful career early in their lives, and have then continued working because their skills are still in demand. But (take my word for it) you're never too old to try something new. Here are some examples of so-called 'late bloomers' – people who have *started* a new career at an advanced stage in their lives.

Grandma Moses, painter – Anna Mary Robertson Moses took up painting in 1935, when she was 75. She had had no formal training, but her paintings were in the tradition of American primitive art. Initially she sold her paintings for a few dollars each, but then she was 'discovered' after a collector saw one of her works in a local shop window. A New York show led to worldwide fame. In 2006 one of her paintings sold for $1.2 million. She went on painting until she died aged 101.

Ronald Reagan, politician – Having worked as a reasonably successful film and TV actor, union leader and corporate spokesman, he was first elected to public office at the age of 55 when he became Governor of California. He went on to become the 40th President of the USA just before his 70th birthday, and served two four-year terms. Not only was he the USA's oldest ever president, but he was regarded by many as one of the most successful of recent times.

Cesar Franck, composer – Born in 1822, Franck worked as a music teacher and an organist in Paris for much of his adult life. He composed various pieces of music in his forties and fifties, but these were not well received. In 1886 (aged 64) he had his first major success with his Violin Sonata. This was followed two years later by his Symphony in D Minor, which was his most successful composition.

Laura Ingalls Wilder, author – Born in 1867, Wilder spent her early years living in log cabins and homesteads in Kansas and Wisconsin, USA. Following a brief career as a schoolteacher, she married and spent the next few decades farming and raising a family. Eventually her daughter encouraged her to write a memoir of her early life. The resulting book, *Pioneer Girl*, was turned down by several publishers. But when she reworked the book at the age of 65, she had more success. It became the first in the hugely successful *Little House on the Prairie* series. Her books went on to be translated into over 40 languages, and sold millions of copies worldwide.

Harlan David Sanders, entrepreneur – Sanders worked in a variety of jobs, including as a farmer, a steamboat pilot and an insurance salesman. When he was 40, he opened a petrol service station and started selling fried chicken to his customers as a sideline. At the age of 65 he opened a restaurant, which he went on to franchise, making him a multi-millionaire. The restaurant was called Kentucky Fried Chicken, and Sanders is now better remembered by the nickname of 'Colonel Sanders'.

So, if you have an unfulfilled ambition or a passion to do something completely new, saying 'I'm too old' is no excuse!

BIOLOGICAL AGE VS ACTUAL AGE

When I go to a school or college reunion I inevitably meet people I haven't seen for a long time – maybe 20, 30 or even 40 years. I find that the old friends or classmates I encounter fall into two groups. There are those I immediately recognise, because I think they 'haven't changed a bit'. And then there will be others who I struggle to recall. Maybe they've got a lot fatter, grown their hair long, become bald, gone grey, grown a beard, shaved off their beard, become heavily tattooed, become wrinkled or started wearing spectacles. Or maybe their faces have simply aged to the extent that they appear to have become different people from the ones I remember.

Some people appear to age quite slowly, while others speed

through their lives. Your biological age, as assessed from a medical point of view, may be very different from your actual age – either higher or lower.

In 2015, researchers from King's College London developed a series of tests to measure a person's biological age. They looked at eighteen indicators of health, including kidney and liver function, blood pressure, cholesterol levels, and the length of a person's telomeres (the protective caps in our chromosomes that prevent DNA damage).[11]

They found a dramatic variation in results. In a group of 38-year-olds, some people had the same physiology as an average 30-year-old, while others had the physiology of a 60-year-old. Although most people in the study had a biological age that was around their real age, some were found to be ageing as fast as three years per chronological year. Others were hardly ageing at all.

King's College London's Dr Andrea Danese explains the significance: 'For the first time, we can see how fast they are ageing. The people who had the oldest biological age were growing old the fastest,' he says. 'With these tests we could detect premature ageing before people begin to develop heart disease, diabetes or dementia – so we could treat them.'[12]

The researchers believe the measurement of biological age will become commonplace. You will simply be assessed by your family doctor on a regular basis and told your biological age. Similarly, health insurance companies and pension providers may start to ask for this information when assessing the premiums or contributions you will be asked to pay.

Apart from undergoing a detailed medical analysis, there are other ways of finding out whether your biological age differs significantly from your actual age. If you go for a medical check-up, you may well be asked to squeeze a handle to measure your hand strength. This usually peaks between the ages of 20 and 40, and then declines slowly after that, and it has been found to be a good indicator of overall muscle strength, as well as an accurate way of predicting disability and mortality.

If you search for 'biological age' online, you'll find a number of tests[13] that claim to measure this by using a variety of lifestyle questions: how much you drink, how much exercise you take, how briskly you walk, and other factors such as how many cars you own (an indicator of wealth – see Chapter 12).

Clearly the concept of biological age has a significant effect on your potential longevity. If your body is biologically already a lot older than your actual age, you are clearly less likely to live a long and healthy life because you will be more susceptible to age-related diseases.

It seems there's an even easier way of measuring how long you are likely to live, according to a study of the population in the UK by two Swedish scientists (published in *The Lancet* in 2015).[14] If you are a middle-aged man and you want to know if you are going to die in the next five years, simply ask yourself how healthy you think you are.

Whether you rate your health as excellent, good, fair or poor is a better predictor of death than any physical measures such as blood pressure and pulse rate. If you feel that you are in excellent health, it probably means that you are.

Recently, I had the pleasure of meeting a remarkable man who bears this theory out.

EVERYTHING IN MODERATION

Heatherslade Residential Home stands in a spectacular seaside location in Southgate, a small village on the Gower Peninsula in South Wales. Its elderly residents appreciate the uninterrupted views of the cliffs and the sea, as well as the chance to spend time in the various seating areas around the gardens.

But this afternoon everyone is looking forward to one of the high points of the week, a visit by Francis Stares (known to locals as Jock), a former dentist turned semi-professional entertainer. As usual, Jock arrives on his trusty Yamaha 125 motor scooter, greets everyone warmly, and then sits down at the piano.

'I just play all the old music hall things – "Down at the Old Bull and Bush" and "My Old Man". When I play, they all sing with gusto,' he says. 'They know all the words – they really enjoy themselves. And that does give me a lot of pleasure because I feel that I've done a little bit of good.'

There's nothing remarkable about that – except that Jock is 101 years old, several years older than all the elderly residents he entertains – and every day (including weekends) he still goes out to work, either travelling on his scooter or in his car, to spread a little happiness in the local community.

Jock welcomed me to his home in Langland, near Swansea, offering me coffee and a plate of his delicious homemade macaroons. He lives surrounded by photos and mementoes that reflect his extraordinary life – as well as the obligatory 100th-birthday card from the Queen. His love of motorbikes began when he was seven years old and his father bought him an 'old banger' from a scrapyard.

'When I'm on my motorbike I feel 20 – I'm just a schoolboy again,' he told me. 'I feel absolutely fantastic on the bike. It's the next best thing to being able to fly because you go through the cool air effortlessly. It's like a drug, really – you become addicted to it. You love that feeling of freedom and the power that you've got under your hands.'

Jock went to Swansea Grammar School, where he was a contemporary of Dylan Thomas. He met his wife Babs in the local post office in 1938, and they worked together at his dentistry practice for 60 years until her death in 2000. After retiring from that profession, he took up his job as a pianist and entertainer.

I have rarely met someone with such an enthusiastic and positive attitude to life. Jock agrees that his cheerful disposition must have played a large part in keeping him active and healthy for so long.

'I have had a very happy life,' he says. 'I had a wonderful childhood and a wonderfully happy marriage with the girl of my dreams. My philosophy is to enjoy life as much as you can. Steer a middle course. Do everything in moderation – eating, drinking, exercise, sex. Don't overdo it.'

DR DAWN'S TOP TIP

Don't fear old age. It doesn't mean an inevitable decline into solitude. There are an increasing number of centenarians living full and active lives. You could be one of them in years to come – and this book will show you how.

CHAPTER 2

THE LUCK
OF THE DICE?

A friend of mine was recently told by his doctor that he had a heart murmur. This means that the doctor heard something unusual in the sound of his heartbeat; the technology used to detect this was nothing more sophisticated than a stethoscope. So, following the doctor's advice, my friend decided to get his heart checked out. An ultrasound scan at the local hospital established that the cause of the heart murmur was a defective heart valve. It's a congenital condition which he must have had all along, but it wasn't detected until he was in his fifties.

'Ah well,' said the cardiologist after reviewing the ultrasound images. 'You can think of it as a gift from your mum and dad!'

We often hear about people who smoke, drink, don't exercise and eat all the wrong foods who live to a very old age. They say that it's just down to having good genes, but the real explanation is probably more simple. For every one of these survivors, there are many more people who lived the same lifestyle and are now dead and buried. And there are many others who are still alive, but who have achieved this through living a healthier lifestyle.

In this chapter I'm going to look at genetic factors that affect how long we live. We all inherit physical attributes – such as the colour of our hair or eyes, our height or weight, or whether we have long fingers that could make us better at playing the piano. So is our lifespan also predetermined by our genes?

Certainly a lot of insurance companies think so. A life insurance application form will often ask at what ages your parents died (if applicable); some will even go back a generation and ask about your grandparents. The assumption is simply that if your ancestors lived to a good age, you're going to be a better bet as a customer because, the longer you live, the less likely it is that they'll need to pay out.

The various centenarians I have met had sharply differing views on the importance of genetics in determining their lifespan. Ann Baer is a prolific writer who still lives in her own home in Richmond, west London; her first book was published when she was 82. She is now 102, but she is adamant that reaching this age had nothing to do with her background.

'People say "Yes, of course it's the genes", she told me. 'But that really isn't true, because I was the second of six children and they're all dead except the first two – my elder sister and myself. I think it's simply a fluke.'

However, the statistics would suggest otherwise. When Ann was born (at the start of World War I), the chance of any person reaching 100 was about 1 in 6,000. So the chance of two consecutive siblings reaching that milestone would be around 1 in 36 million. Still simply a fluke?

The 'nature versus nurture' debate is as old as science itself. Is everything about us foretold by genetic destiny, or is it due to the effects of our environment and personal experience? As you would expect, the answer lies somewhere in between. However, it's important to know exactly how our genetic make-up determines our lives and our lifespans – then we can discover what biological hand nature has dealt us, and what (if anything) we can do about it. More importantly, we can take control of all the other non-genetic lifestyle factors that we know can make a difference.

THE GENE GENIES

To understand how we become the people we are, we need to know a bit about our DNA. This is an abbreviation for deoxyribonucleic acid. It's a long molecule that contains every person's unique genetic code. DNA is like an instruction manual that tells every part of your body how to develop, live and reproduce.

Every creature on earth is programmed by their DNA. We're not all that different from some of our animal relatives – for example, humans and chimpanzees share a remarkable 98.8% of the same DNA. (This is because our species are thought to have evolved from a common ancestor, with the split taking place about seven million years ago.)

Although DNA was discovered in 1869 by Friedrich Miescher, a German scientist, its real importance was not understood until 1953 when the British-based team of Francis Crick and James Watson published their famous paper showing how DNA's 'double helix' structure carried biological information. A third man, Maurice Wilkins, was also credited with contributing to the research, and the three men were awarded the Nobel Prize in Medicine in 1962. A fourth scientist, Rosalind Franklin, was recognised posthumously for helping to make this discovery; sadly, she died at the age of 37, probably as a direct result of having worked extensively with X-rays in her research. More recently biologists from all over the world collaborated on the Human Genome Project to show exactly how human DNA is structured. This project was successfully completed in 2003.

Your personal DNA is what makes you 'you', and (unless you have an identical twin) it's unique. DNA molecules are very long, so they are tightly coiled to form structures called chromosomes. Humans have 23 pairs of chromosomes in the nucleus of every cell – one chromosome is inherited from your father, and one from your mother. One pair of chromosomes also determines your sex. You get an X-chromosome from your mother and either an X- or a

Y-chromosome from your father. If the result is XX, you are female; the XY combination makes you male. (A few people are born with just one sex chromosome, and some may have three or more.)

Even though your DNA is extremely complex, it's very easy to copy, and this is what happens all the time. Every time your body makes a new cell, that cell contains a new copy of your DNA. For example, your body gets a whole new coating of skin cells every six weeks. Each of those new cells has the exact same DNA.

As we get older, the process by which your body makes new cells becomes less efficient. At the ends of your chromosomes, there are sections of DNA called telomeres, which protect your genetic data. These telomeres have been compared to the plastic tips on shoelaces, because they protect the chromosome ends from fraying. But each time a cell divides, these telomeres get shorter. When a telomere becomes too short, the chromosome reaches a critical length and can no longer be copied. This is the process of ageing. That's why a lot of research is being carried out to find ways that these telomeres can be repaired or lengthened, as this could have a dramatic effect on slowing down the ageing process.

Because your DNA is unique, it's very easy to identify an individual using DNA profiling (also known as genetic fingerprinting). You can have a paternity test to determine whether two individuals are biologically a parent and their child. Also, DNA profiling is widely used in police investigations to establish whether or not a particular individual was at the scene of a crime. In each case all you need is a very small tissue sample, since every cell contains the information you need.

So how does your DNA affect your lifespan? There are three ways in which this can happen:

Bad genes – You inherit certain genetic variations that make it more likely that you will at some stage contract a fatal disease, such as a particular type of cancer.

Good genes – You are somewhat luckier and inherit a set of genes that makes your body more resistant to a particular disease, giving you a genetic advantage.

Genetic disorders – The genes themselves are the cause of a serious illness or condition that could be obvious at birth, or which may manifest itself later in life.

COMMON GENETIC DISORDERS

Although science has identified very many different genetic disorders, most are quite rare, affecting one person in several thousand or even million. They may be hereditary, passed down from one of your parents' genes – although in many cases that parent may themselves be completely unaffected – or the disorder may simply arise because your DNA has been damaged or mutated in some way. This could be totally random, or it may be a result of exposure to some adverse environmental factor. For example, if pregnant women are exposed to high doses of radiation, their children are more likely to get cancer. (This was confirmed by research into the victims of the atomic bombs in Hiroshima and Nagasaki.)

Examples of some of the more common genetic disorders are listed below.

Cystic fibrosis: This is one of the most common inherited diseases in the Western world. Caused by a mutation in one particular gene, cystic fibrosis makes the body's mucus excessively thick and sticky, leading to blockages within the lungs and airways. Over time, this causes severe breathing problems. Many people are a carrier of cystic fibrosis but have no symptoms themselves. However, they can pass on the faulty gene to their children: if a child inherits a faulty gene from both parents, he or she will have the disease. Although there is no cure for cystic fibrosis, treatments have improved greatly in recent years. The average life expectancy of someone with cystic fibrosis is 41, although this figure is likely to improve significantly in the next few years.

Sickle cell anaemia: This is an inherited disorder of the haemoglobin in blood. The red blood cells become abnormally shaped, which restricts blood flow. Sickle cell anaemia is disproportionately common in Africans and African Americans. It is possible to diagnose the condition in a child before it is born. Symptoms include chronic fatigue, pneumonia, inflammation of the joints, and occasional bouts of acute pain. The most common cause of death is bacterial infection. Globally many children die from sickle cell anaemia before they are three, and overall life expectancies are about 25 years lower than for the general population.

Down's syndrome: Also known as Down syndrome, this genetic disorder is caused by the presence of all or part of a third copy of one particular chromosome, chromosome 21. These extra genes lead to changes in development of the embryo, resulting in distinctive physical abnormalities. People with Down's syndrome also have learning disabilities, but the level of disability varies widely from one person to another. According to recent NHS figures, around 1 in 1,000 children is born with this condition. As for life expectancy, there has been a dramatic improvement over the past century. A child born with Down's syndrome 100 years ago would only have lived to the age of nine. Now the life expectancy is typically 50–60 years, with many people reaching their 80s.

Pregnant women often ask me about the various tests they can have for Down's syndrome. I would always recommend getting these tests, as you can then make a decision based on the information available. All pregnant women in the UK are routinely offered the so-called combined test, which involves a blood test and an ultrasound scan. This test cannot tell you for certain whether your baby will have Down's syndrome. (When I was pregnant with my first child, I was told there was a 10% chance that my baby would have Down's.) If you are told your baby is at high risk, you can then choose to have a further diagnostic test, such as an amniocentesis. This involves taking a small amount of fluid from the amniotic sac that surrounds the developing foetus. It carries a small risk of causing a miscarriage, but it will tell you for certain whether or not your baby has the condition. A safer and more accurate test has recently been introduced in the UK – the non-invasive prenatal test is a simple blood test that replaces the combined test, but you may still need an amniocentesis to get a 100% accurate result.

THREE-PARENT BABIES

There are many other genetic disorders, including serious conditions such as Duchenne Muscular Dystrophy, haemophilia, and Canavan disease. Others, such as colour-blindness, are relatively harmless and have no impact on life expectancy. In most cases there is no way of preventing the disorder if the defective gene is present – but this situation is beginning to change.

Leigh's disease is a disorder that affects the central nervous system. It's caused by a defect in the mother's mitochondria, often described as the power plant of the body's cells. Recently Sharon Bernardi from Sunderland in the north-east of England lost all seven of her children to this disease. She felt fine during each pregnancy, and the births went well, but then things started to go wrong. Her first three children died within hours of being born, and at first no one knew why. It then emerged that Sharon's mother had suffered three stillbirths before Sharon was born.

'I didn't know about my mum's history,' Sharon said. 'There

was no need for me to know. I was my mother's only child and I think that in her era people didn't really talk about things like they do now.'[1]

Further investigation revealed that members of Sharon's extended family had lost another eight children in this way. Then along came Edward, Sharon's fourth child. Although his health was often poor, he was a cheerful, active boy. At the age of four he started to have seizures, and it was then that doctors were finally able to diagnose the problem. Edward died at the age of 21. Sharon had three more babies but, tragically, they all died before they were two years old.

In 2017 there was a lot of publicity about the sad case of Charlie Gard, who had a rare inherited disease called infantile onset encephalomyopathy mitochondrial DNA depletion syndrome (MDDS). When he was born, Charlie appeared completely normal. But about a month later his parents noticed that he was having trouble lifting his head. This is because MDDS causes muscle weakness. Further genetic and clinical tests confirmed the diagnosis. There is no cure for MDDS. Charlie died just before his first birthday.

Such diseases are extremely rare, but in future it may become possible to avoid them. You may have read about 'three-parent babies' in the press. This refers to a pioneering technique to prevent babies being born with a range of mitochondrial diseases such as Leigh's. In this procedure, the vast majority of a baby's DNA comes from the mother and father, but a small amount also comes from a third person – a female donor who does not carry the defect. However, this technique is still in the very early stages, as the UK's fertility watchdog only approved it at the end of 2016.

KNOWLEDGE IS POWER

The genetic disorders we've looked at so far are easy to identify: if you're born with a particular genetic defect, you *will* get the disease

or condition. Things get more complicated when we look at diseases
in which a genetic disorder may be only part of the story. These are
called polygenic disorders – where the condition is likely to be
associated with the effects of multiple genes, in combination with
lifestyle and environmental factors.

Heart disease is a good example. If you have a family history of
cardiovascular disease, you have an increased risk of developing a
disease such as angina, heart attack, heart failure or stroke. If both
your parents suffered from heart disease before they were 55, your
chance of developing it yourself before this age is increased by about
50% compared to the general population. (We'll return to this in
Chapter 7.)

Other diseases that have been shown to have a genetic
component include Alzheimer's disease, high blood pressure, diabetes,
arthritis and various types of cancer, including breast cancer.

DR DAWN'S TOP TIP

Find out as much as you can about your family's medical history. You
probably already know a lot about your first-degree relatives
(parents, brothers and sisters). I suggest you do some research into
second-degree relatives (grandparents, aunts, uncles, etc.). Knowing
your family medical history gives you the chance to reduce your
own risk. For example, if patients have an inherited risk of certain
cancers, I might recommend more frequent screening, usually starting
at an earlier age.

In 2013 the actress Angelina Jolie, then aged 37, had both breasts
surgically removed after finding out that she carries a genetic
mutation of the BRCA1 gene, one that dramatically increases the
chance of being diagnosed with potentially fatal breast cancer. The
mutation suggested she had an 87% risk of getting breast cancer and
a 50% risk of ovarian cancer. She had already lost her mother, her
grandmother and her aunt to cancer.

Writing in the *New York Times* after the operation, Jolie said: 'I went through what I imagine thousands of other women have felt. I told myself to stay calm, to be strong, and that I had no reason to think I wouldn't live to see my children grow up and to meet my grandchildren.'[2]

Two years later Angelina Jolie underwent further surgery to have her ovaries removed. Her decision to have the operations – and also to go public about them – has had a significant effect on raising awareness about the potentially fatal BRCA1 gene. The 'Jolie effect' has resulted in far more women having the test (even though it can cost around £2,500).[3]

'It is not easy to make these decisions,' Jolie said. 'But it is possible to take control and tackle head-on any health issue. You can seek advice, learn about the options, and make choices that are right for you. Knowledge is power.'

But you can only make choices if you have that knowledge. What happened to the late broadcaster Sir David Frost is a cautionary tale. Sir David died from a heart attack in 2013 when he was 74. His post-mortem revealed that he had a genetic condition called hypertrophic cardiomyopathy (HCM), which can cause a thickening of the heart wall, which in turn can cause sudden death at any age. But, for whatever reason, this information was not passed on to his family. Two years later one of his three sons, 31-year-old Miles Frost, collapsed and died from HCM while out jogging. One of his surviving brothers, Wilf, said: 'If you'd seen him the day before he died everyone would have said Miles is looking so good – so fit and so healthy. [It was] a ticking time bomb in the whole family.'[4]

It is always good to hear when something good comes out of bad. The remaining brothers have set up a charity to raise awareness of this inherited condition, which will work to avoid some of these premature deaths in the future.

If you have HCM, there's a 50% chance that your children will inherit it. But with proper treatment, including the use of drugs and sometimes a pacemaker, it's possible to control it so that you can lead a normal life.

SEND IN THE CLONES

Apart from identifying certain genes that are linked to the risk of serious diseases, is there a genetic basis for longevity itself? Professor Stuart Kim from Stanford University in California is one of the leading experts in this field. He believes he has identified four specific genes that are linked to living an exceptionally long life. 'There's a reasonably strong genetic component to becoming a centenarian,' he says. 'We're beginning to unravel the mystery of why some people age so successfully compared to the normal population.'[5]

Professor Kim's team searched for these longevity genes in a group of about 800 people aged 100 or over. They then compared the results with a control group of people who were elderly, but not quite as old. For example, the study found that a genetic variation associated with having type O blood was more common in centenarians. In other words, if you're type O, you're more likely to make it to 100!

In Chapter 1 I told you about the apparent difference between actual age and biological age. According to another piece of research, it seems the speed at which we age may be linked to our DNA. This is known as our 'epigenetic clock'.

'We are often struck by the difference between our patients' chronological age and how old they appear physiologically,' says Professor Douglas Kiel of the Harvard Medical School, where this research is taking place.[6] His team looked at the DNA of over 13,000 people and compared it to how well they had aged. They found that an unlucky 5% of the population age at a much faster rate than average. These people were found to be 50% more likely to die at any age. In other words, some people are destined to age faster and die younger – regardless of how they treat their bodies.

There is a genetic condition called Hutchinson–Gilford syndrome that causes people to age at about ten times the normal rate. Even when only 6–12 months old, a baby with this disease will begin to show visible signs of ageing, including thinning skin, wrinkles and greying hair. The average life expectancy for someone with this disease is around 13 years; most sufferers die from heart disease. Fortunately, this condition is extremely rare, occurring in about 1 in 8 million children.

As I mentioned earlier, life insurance companies believe there is a strong link between parental longevity and offspring longevity, but of course that doesn't necessarily mean that the link is entirely genetic. Parents not only pass on their genes; they also pass on patterns of behaviour.

An obvious example is smoking. If parents smoke, their child is likely to be exposed to secondary smoke during their early life. It is also more likely that the children will themselves become smokers. Both generations are likely to die well before they should, but it doesn't have anything to do with genetics. Conversely, parents can instil good habits in their children, teaching them about the benefits of exercise and a healthy diet. Again there will be a link between the longevity of the two generations, but this is more down to learned lifestyle than DNA.

Other evidence about the genetic basis for longevity is based on studying identical twins. In the UK about one in every 67 pregnancies results in multiple births (usually twins, but occasionally triplets, quadruplets or more). Most twins are non-identical (or dizygotic) – they begin to grow in the womb after two separate eggs are fertilised by two separate sperm. Women are more likely to give birth to twins if there's a family history of multiple births on your mother's side. The chance of a multiple pregnancy increases as women get older too.

Identical or monozygotic twins are completely different. Here an egg is fertilised, begins to develop, and then splits in two. The reason this happens is unknown – there certainly isn't a genetic factor. You could say having identical twins is just a piece of good luck (although it can get very expensive when you're buying two prams, cots and all the other baby equipment!). About a third of twins are identical twins.

Scientists get very excited about identical twins. Why? Because, as I've already mentioned, they have exactly the same DNA. This means they are clones, born with exactly the same physical characteristics. By following the progress of these twins through their lives, doctors can try to assess which health-related factors are genetic and which factors are environmental.

In some cases identical twins are separated at birth (for example, if they are adopted by different families). By observing what happens to them later in life, it becomes possible to track the influence of environmental factors more clearly, and then work out how 'heritable' a particular trait may be. For example, a long-term study in Denmark[7] found that if one identical twin died of a stroke, there was an 18% chance that the other one would also die of a stroke. This is about double the figure for the general population, and it indicates that heredity does play a part in the likelihood of having a stroke. But you can look at this another way: if one twin has a stroke, there is a less than 20% chance that the other one will. This suggests that around 80% of the risk is associated with environmental factors.

In the case of coronary heart disease (CHD), the genetic factor is even stronger. Another study (this time carried out in Sweden[8]) found that if one male identical twin died of CHD, there was a 57% chance that the other twin would die of the same cause. For female identical twins, the figure was lower, at 38%. But if you need proof that genetics can play a part, here it is.

SHOULD YOU HAVE GENETIC TESTING?

Type 'genetic testing' into a search engine and you'll find dozens of companies that offer a simple, discreet analysis of your DNA. You don't need to go to a clinic. You just send them a small sample of your saliva and the results will be emailed to you within a few weeks. Prices vary from about £70 to over £2,000, depending on the nature and complexity of what they offer.

Some of these services will give you information about your family background. For example, they can tell you in which countries your ancestors probably lived. Some people have used these DNA tests to track down close relatives with whom they had lost contact or who they had never known. You'll also be given data about your physical traits – the test may identify lactose intolerance, the tendency to have freckles, a propensity for male pattern baldness, or your sensitivity to pain. Much of this information may be interesting, but of limited value.

The health information is slightly more complicated. Typically genetic tests will tell you about possible health risks and inherited conditions. This includes information about genetic variants, so you can see if you may be the carrier of certain diseases or deficiencies – even if you don't have the problem yourself.

I had one of these tests myself a couple of years ago. The test I had specialised in providing dietary and fitness information. I discovered that I have a high sensitivity to carbohydrates, so I should cut down dramatically on foods such as bread to avoid putting on weight. It also recommended that I should eat higher than average amounts of fish oil and vitamin D. On the fitness front, the DNA test concluded that I have a 'higher than average risk of sports-related soft tissue injury'. In other words, I need to be careful when doing certain types of sport or exercise.

So should you consider having a genetic test? I think it may be advisable if you or your family has a known history of a certain disease. It could then help you to make choices about how to manage your health, and it could be a factor in deciding whether or not to have children. But any test is, of course, voluntary, and making a decision about whether or not to have one can be complex.

DR DAWN'S TOP TIP

You should treat the results of any genetic testing with caution. These tests cannot tell you everything about inherited diseases. A positive result does not always mean you will develop a particular disease.

In some instances genetic tests have been carried out posthumously. In 2014 researchers for a Channel 4 documentary analysed samples of hair from the late Elvis Presley. The singer, who died at the age of 42, was already known to have had an irregular heartbeat, high blood pressure and bad eyesight. Many people blamed his early death on his fondness for junk food. But the DNA test suggested that he may have died because of genetic conditions that made him unusually prone to obesity and heart disease. Of course, if he had known this, he might have chosen to adapt his lifestyle accordingly before it was too late.

CONGENITAL DISORDERS

Even if your genetic background is favourable, there's still plenty that can go wrong before a baby makes it into the outside world. It's estimated that one out of every 33 babies has a congenital disorder – a structural deformity in some part of the body that exists at the time he or she is born. It could be caused by adverse factors when the baby is developing in the womb.

If a mother-to-be drinks too much during pregnancy (particularly during the early stages), the baby may have foetal alcohol syndrome. The UK has one of the highest incidences of this in the world. About 40% of British mothers-to-be drink during pregnancy, and the condition is thought to affect about at least 1 in every 100 babies.[9] Foetal alcohol syndrome can cause the baby to be intellectually impaired, or to develop heart or kidney disease later in life. Foetal alcohol syndrome is notoriously hard to track or diagnose, because women are reluctant to admit they have been drinking during pregnancy. Furthermore, a lot of women are unaware that they are pregnant in the early stages: by the time they give up, it could be too late for the foetus.

As you might expect, smoking and the use of certain drugs during pregnancy have also been shown to cause congenital disorders. Various drugs can cause birth defects, including illegal ones (such as cocaine) and others taken for medicinal purposes, including isotretinoin (an acne drug), lithium, high doses of vitamin A, some antibiotics and warfarin (the blood-thinning drug). The most notorious example of a drug that caused birth defects is thalidomide.

In some parts of the world (such as South East Asia, South and Central America), similar problems have been caused in the past three years by the mother's exposure to the Zika virus. This virus is mainly spread by mosquitoes and causes only mild symptoms in most adults, but it has been linked to serious birth defects, in particular the tendency for babies to be born with very small heads (microcephaly).

At the start of this chapter I mentioned a friend with a congenital heart disorder. This is actually quite common, and occurs in about 1 in 110 births. But you may live through several decades – or even the whole of your life – without realising you have a potentially serious condition. Fortunately, most heart defects can be corrected, or at least improved, by surgery or the use of drugs.

A GENETICALLY MODIFIED FUTURE

In most cases the genes you're born with are the genes you'll live with all your life. There's not much you can do to change them – yet. But as well as recent progress with mitochondrial diseases, a lot of research is under way to find ways of replacing other types of faulty gene with healthy ones. Some of this research involves the use of viruses. So, for example, it could be possible to develop viruses that can get into the body's cells and introduce new DNA (that is, after all, what viruses do).

Scientists have already been able to create genetically modified (GM) mice that can have their lifespan extended by up to 35%. This research involves removing senescent (worn-out) cells that accumulate with age and have a destructive effect on the body. These cells are closely associated with age-related diseases and frailty. A team at the Mayo Clinic in Minnesota created a strain of mouse with a 'suicide gene' that targets and kills these cells when activated by a drug.

'All the mice that were treated to remove their senescent cells had a lifespan extension from 25% to 35%,' said Dr Darren Baker, who was in charge of the research. 'In all cases there is a significant health and lifespan extension.'[10]

But it may be a long time before this sort of research can be applied to human beings – not least because of ethical issues. Most countries have not yet introduced legislation to control genetic modification in human reproduction, but all those that have legislation have banned it. There is also a practical problem. Because people live a lot longer than mice, it would take decades before we found out if such techniques have actually had a significant effect on extending our lives – or what other implications there could be.

Future generations are also likely to take a more interventionist approach to conceiving children. At the moment it's usually a matter of luck, with one of several possible eggs waiting in the womb for whichever sperm happens to win the race to get there first. People can – in theory – choose some factors affecting the genes they want to pass on to their children ('designer babies'). But this is very rare – and very controversial.[11]

Up to now, these so-called 'designer babies' have been the stuff of science fiction. But one day you could be able to choose exactly what characteristics you want your baby to have – and you will be able to select genes that are free from disease, and which will give your child the best chance of living a very long life. Few would argue with that logic, but where would you draw the line? It would be possible to choose the sex of your next child, or the colour of their hair, but should that be allowed to happen?

IT'S NOT JUST GENETICS

So is your lifespan just down to luck? If you really thought that, you probably wouldn't be reading this book. Good genes *do* help to determine how long you'll live and how healthy you will be, but lifestyle choices generally make a bigger difference. The older you get, the more your destiny depends on how you live than on your genes.

A series of studies of twins in Norway and Sweden concluded that somewhere between 20% and 30% of the overall variation in lifespans is caused by genetic differences. However, Dr James Vaupel of the impressively named Laboratory of Survival and Longevity in Rostock, Germany, thinks the genetic influence is much less. In an article in *The New York Times* (31 August 2016), he argued:

> *How tall your parents are compared to the average height explains 80–90% of how tall you are compared to the average person. Only 3% of how long you live compared to the average person can be explained by how long your parents lived. You*

really learn very little about your own life span from your parents' life spans. That's what the evidence shows. Even twins, identical twins, die at different times.[12]

On average, Dr Vaupel said, identical twins die more than ten years apart.

The most obvious proof that lifestyle counts for much more than genes comes from taking another look at the various statistics in Chapter 1. People's life expectancy has rocketed. On average we're living twice as long as people did only a century ago. But there's no evidence that the human race has fundamentally changed in this period: our DNA is structurally very similar to that of our recent ancestors. Human evolution takes a lot longer.

Of course, much of this improvement in life expectancy is down to medicine. A lot of diseases that killed people in the past are now completely survivable. One in fifteen people gets appendicitis, a disease that was once 100% fatal. In fact, that's what killed my aunt at the tender age of six. When I developed appendicitis many decades later, I had a relatively minor operation and was out of hospital in days.

It's the way we live, and the lifestyle choices we make, that will primarily decide our fate.

DR DAWN'S TOP TIP

If you're unfit, overweight or chronically unhealthy, blaming it on your 'bad genes' isn't going to fool anyone. You need to take control and do something to improve your chances of living a longer, healthier life. How can you achieve this? Read the next chapter to find out.

Chapter 3
CIGARETTES AND ALCOHOL

It will come as no shock to you that a book advising you how to live a long and healthy life will, at some point, be tackling cigarettes and alcohol, and it won't be any surprise that I have decided to talk about these issues early on in this book. There is good reason for this. I'd like to start with smoking.

If you're not a smoker, you may be tempted to skip this chapter. Please don't. It contains some shocking facts that you could drop into conversation over the dinner table to prevent your kids from ever wanting to smoke.

SMOKING

Although smoking has reduced in the UK since the introduction of the smoking ban in 2007, smoking is still responsible for 96,000 deaths in the UK every year. On average, a lifelong smoker will lose at least ten years from their life, and is more likely to have a poor quality of life in their later years. To achieve our goal of living well to 101 years, smoking has got to be a no-no. The fact is, about half of all lifelong smokers will die of their habit. My dear grandad was one – he smoked all his life and died aged 63 of lung cancer. Sadly, his father died at the same age of a smoking-related illness. I suspect the fact that I have never smoked has more to do with losing him when I was young than anything else. He was a wonderful grandparent. Most people know that smoking increases the risk of developing lung cancer, which sadly has a poorer prognosis than many other types of cancer. Of men diagnosed with lung cancer, 30% will survive a year; women fare slightly better at 35%, and that means that around two-thirds of people with lung cancer die within a year of diagnosis. Smoking is responsible for 80% of deaths from lung cancer. In fact, more than a quarter of all cancer deaths can be linked to smoking. These include cancer of the mouth, throat, oesophagus, stomach, pancreas, liver, bladder, kidney and cervix.

SO WHERE DID IT ALL START?

It is generally accepted that Sir Walter Raleigh first brought tobacco from Virginia to England on 27 July 1586. According to the history books, it is likely that tobacco reached our shores sooner, and could have been brought here as early as 1565. One of the things I love about medicine is that we are always learning, and back in those days it was thought that smoking tobacco was good for you. It was even hailed as a treatment for cancer!

Things changed quickly, and at the turn of the seventeenth century, there were already concerns about the potential health risks associated with smoking – but that didn't stop its inexorable rise in popularity. In 1638, three million pounds of Virginia tobacco was sent to England, rising rapidly to 25 million pounds by 1680.

When the plague arrived in the UK in 1665, smoking tobacco was seen as a way of clearing the air, and people were so convinced of its benefits that public schoolboys at Eton College were made to smoke a pipe at breakfast, to help keep the air clean and reduce the risks of contracting the plague!

WHERE ARE WE TODAY?

Close to one in five British adults now smokes (19%), with slightly more men (20%) than women (17%) enjoying the habit, which equates to 9.6 million adults smoking in the UK. This is a massive reduction on recent years. Smoking has more than halved since 1974, when 51% of men and 41% of women were regular smokers. We have a long way to go – two-thirds of smokers start before the age of eighteen and, of those who try smoking, between a third and a half will become regular smokers. If you are reading this book for *you*, but have teenage children, it may be an idea to leave the book open at this chapter!

DR DAWN'S TOP TIP

Young people are still taking up smoking – it's easier never to start than it is to quit, so make sure the young people around you know all the facts.

WHAT IS IN A CIGARETTE?

Nicotine is the addictive component of a cigarette. When nicotine is inhaled, it reaches the brain in six seconds. However, it's not the nicotine that kills you, it's the thousands of other toxins contained in a cigarette that cause the harm. A single cigarette contains over 4,000 chemicals, either as gases or as minute particles. More than 50 of these chemicals are carcinogenic – they are known to cause cancer. Some of them are highly toxic, including:

- arsenic – used in rat poison
- carbon monoxide – released in car exhaust fumes
- cyanide – used in pesticides
- benzene – found in rubber cement

- toluene – used to manufacture paint
- formaldehyde – used as an embalming fluid
- acetone – found in nail varnish remover
- butane – used in lighter fuel
- cadmium – found in battery acid
- lead – used in batteries
- tar – used for road surfaces.

It makes horrific reading, doesn't it? Why would you want to put any of those compounds into your body? But that's what 9.6 million Brits do several times every day. It's not difficult to see how exposing yourself to those toxins on a regular basis is going to have a negative impact, not only on your longevity, but also your general health and well-being.

Filters were added to cigarettes in the 1950s, when we started to learn about the health hazards associated with smoking, and it was thought that adding a filter would trap some of the tar and toxic particles in cigarette smoke and reduce the health risks. Studies have shown that low-tar cigarettes are often also low in nicotine, and people smoking them tend to compensate for the reduction in nicotine by smoking more, in the false belief that low-tar cigarettes are safer. It has been illegal to describe one brand of cigarette as safer than another, by using terms such as *light* or *mild*, since 2003.

DR DAWN'S TOP TIP

Next time you reach for a cigarette, take the list of chemicals with you and imagine yourself licking tarmac, chewing on rubber cement or drinking a cocktail of battery acid, lighter fuel and nail varnish remover. Maybe that cigarette won't be quite so appealing!

WHAT ABOUT PASSIVE SMOKING?

Passive smoking is when we breathe in other people's smoke and that includes the smoke that is exhaled by smokers and sidestream smoke – which is the smoke constantly emitted from a lit cigarette. The toxic gases in sidestream smoke are higher in concentration because they have not been inhaled, leaving some toxins behind in the smoker's lungs. It is thought that as much as 85% of the smoke in a room is due to sidestream smoke, and this causes short- and long-term health problems. In the short term, most people will be familiar with the symptoms of eye and throat irritation, coughing, and possibly even headaches and nausea when in a smoky room. Long-term health effects are more worrying, and were influential in drawing up the smoking ban in 2007 (when the UK government passed a new law making it illegal for anyone to smoke in an enclosed public place and within a workplace). The International Agency for Research on Cancer conducted a review of the evidence on passive smoking and cancer in 2002, and concluded that exposure to second-hand smoke increases the risk of lung cancer in non-smokers by 20–30% and the risk of coronary heart disease by 25–35%. One in eight patients who develops lung cancer has never smoked a single cigarette, and it's generally accepted that passive smoking plays a huge role here. Children are particularly vulnerable to the effects of second-hand smoke. The Royal College of Physicians estimates that nearly 10,000 children are admitted to hospital every year due to passive smoking and that, every year, second-hand smoke accounts for:

- over 20,000 lower respiratory tract infections
- 120,000 middle ear infections
- 22,000 attacks of wheezing or asthma
- 200 cases of bacterial meningitis
- 40 cot deaths (that's 20% of all cot deaths each year).

If you can't give up for yourself, maybe you should think about the impact your smoking has on those around you.

Remember, the smoke from one cigarette stays in a room (even with the window open) for at least a couple of hours.

When I was working on a TV show called *Embarrassing Bodies*, I remember doing a road show in Scarborough one weekend – we were focusing on the health effects of smoking. I had a hand-held machine called a spirometer, which measures lung function. I asked smokers to blow into the machine, entered their age, and the machine calculated the age of their lungs. I met one man who had been a heavy smoker all his life. He was 55, but according to my machine, his lungs were nearer those of an 80-year-old. I thought that would frighten him, but he seemed unfazed by the news. I then asked his wife, who had never smoked in her life, to use the machine. She was 50, and according to my machine, her lungs were those of a 65-year-old. His face totally changed: he had tears in his eyes. He swore to me that he would make an appointment to see his GP the following Monday, and would make sure he stopped smoking. I'd love to know how he got on – I'm hopeful he succeeded. Sometimes, what we can't do for ourselves, we can do for those who mean the most to us – and that could even include your pets! A study in America showed that even limited exposure to cigarette smoke more than doubled a cat's risk of developing feline lymphoma,[1] and other studies have shown a link between second-hand smoke and cancer in dogs.

DR DAWN'S TOP TIP

If you are smoking around others, always try to smoke outside. If you must smoke inside, don't leave your cigarette burning unnecessarily. If you have had enough, put it out.

CAN I SMOKE IN MY CAR?

It has been illegal in England and Wales to smoke in a car when children are present since October 2015. The reasoning behind this is that second-hand smoke is even more concentrated in such a restricted environment. Research from Canada[2] showed that a single cigarette smoked in a stationary car, with the windows closed, results in a concentration of second-hand smoke eleven times higher than in a bar where smoking was permitted! Even opening the window won't negate the effect – with the windows open, and the fan on high, the level of second-hand smoke in a car produced by a single cigarette is around two-thirds the level found in a smokers' bar – not exactly an environment in which you want your children to spend time.

ARE E-CIGARETTES HEALTHIER?

I am a fan of e-cigarettes. I know they have had some adverse press, but the bottom line is that they are safer than the real thing. I have already said that it isn't the nicotine that kills you, and e-cigarettes are designed to deliver pharmaceutically pure nicotine, without the other toxins that cause so much harm. I believe that e-cigarettes should be regulated, and produced in factories adhering to industry standards – at the time of writing, the wheels are in motion for this to be a legal requirement in the UK. I encourage my patients to try them if they are interested. For some patients, they are an effective way of reducing nicotine intake – some of my patients don't want to give up smoking altogether, and I would rather they got their nicotine hit from an e-cigarette than a traditional one.

Some people have also voiced concerns that e-cigarettes could become a gateway drug for young people who may be at risk of starting smoking properly. This is certainly something we should keep an eye on, but there is no evidence for this – and I think I know why. When cigarettes were first launched on the social scene, they had a glamorous, sexy image, but if you watch someone smoking an e-cigarette today, they usually hold it in the palm of the hand and the action of inhaling is furtive. I think it's important that we don't allow advertising to change that image and make it look cool to smoke e-cigarettes. If that were to happen, I would be concerned that non-smokers would be encouraged to take up the habit.

WHAT ARE THE HEALTH RISKS ASSOCIATED WITH SMOKING?

Each year, around 36,000 people die from lung cancer in the UK and, as I have said, most of those deaths are related to smoking. That leaves over 60,000 smoking-related deaths not linked to lung cancer. Let me give you some frightening statistics:

- Smokers under the age of 40 have a five times greater risk of having a heart attack than non-smokers.
- Women who smoke are likely to go through menopause on average two years earlier, increasing their risk of osteoporosis.
- Smoking is a major cause of impotence in men and increases the production of abnormal sperm.
- Over 37,000 people die each year of other cancers caused by smoking.
- Smoking causes around 1,800 stomach ulcers each year, half of which are fatal.
- Over 16,000 people die each year from vascular disease caused by smoking.
- 25,000 people die each year from chronic lung diseases, such as emphysema, caused by smoking.
- About 12% of all cases of type 2 diabetes can be attributed to smoking.

I'd like to talk about those figures, because the fatalities are the tip of the iceberg. Thousands of people are living their later years with no quality of life because they are desperately short of breath. My dad's best friend was a vibrant man, full of life – as a young child, I remember him being so active – but he died prematurely because of his smoking habit. In the years before his death, I remember him sitting in a chair, even unable to walk to the kitchen to make a cup of tea. He was literally a shadow of the man I had known, and that image still haunts me.

DR DAWN'S TOP TIP

If you get the opportunity to talk to a smoker who has developed lung disease as a result of their smoking, please take it. My patients who have developed Chronic Obstructive Pulmonary Disaese (COPD) all tell me they wish they had never started smoking. I'm sure their stories will help put you off the habit too.

HOW CAN I GIVE UP SMOKING?

I've given you plenty of reasons to give up but I do appreciate that giving up smoking is hard. Nicotine is highly addictive and most of the people I have met over the years who have managed to finally quit the habit make several attempts before succeeding. A survey of smoking-related behaviour and attitudes[3] found that one in four smokers had attempted to quit in the previous year, and one in five had made three attempts in the previous year. Don't let that put you off trying – the more times you have tried, the more likely you are to be successful, so stay focused.

The other thing to consider is that quitting with support has been shown time and time again to improve success rates. You are four times more likely to quit for good with help. The NHS offers free smoking cessation services and your local surgery will be able to refer you to your nearest clinic. When you enrol, you may attend sessions for a couple of weeks before you start to give up smoking, and this allows you to identify your weaknesses, helps you to prepare, and gives you the best chance of success. Your smoking cessation advisor will also be able to talk you through all the various prescription medicines available to help you stop smoking. These include:

- **Champix (varenicicline)** – this is available on prescription to patients aged over 18. It works by reducing cravings and the effects you feel if you smoke a cigarette. You start taking it a couple of weeks before your quit date. You usually then take it for a further ten weeks while you give up.
- **Zyban (bupropion hydrochloride)** – another prescription pill that you start a couple of weeks before your quit date and continue for a couple of months.
- **Nicotine gum** – this is available in two strengths, 2 milligrams (mg) for those who smoke less than 20 a day and 4 mg for heavier smokers. When you chew the gum, you will notice a hot taste as the nicotine is released. You can then place the gum inside your cheek until the sensation fades, or you feel you need more nicotine, and then you can chew again to release more nicotine. You will need to replace the gum when chewing no longer provides that sensation (suggesting that there is no more nicotine in the gum).
- **Nicotine patches** – patches can be worn for 24 hours at a time or for 16 hours while you are awake. They work by slowly releasing nicotine directly into the bloodstream. They come in different strengths, and your smoking cessation advisor will decide which strength you need depending on how many cigarettes you smoke. This is a time to be honest with yourself and your advisor so that you start on the correct dose and give yourself the best chance of success.

- **Nicotine lozenges** – these work in a similar way to gum, but should be sucked for 20 to 30 minutes until they dissolve. Over the weeks, you should need to use the lozenges less frequently.
- **Nicotine inhalators** – these are quite useful for those who miss doing something with their hands, as they mimic the act of smoking as well as delivering the required nicotine. Each inhalator contains about 400 puffs.
- **Nicotine nasal spray** – the lining of the nose is an effective surface for absorption. Using a nasal spray will give a quick burst of nicotine. It is the fastest way (other than smoking) of getting nicotine to the brain and it can be a useful tool for hardened smokers.
- **Nicotine microtabs** – these dissolve under the tongue and can be used initially every hour, with the aim of gradually reducing the dose.

When you attend a smoking cessation clinic, you will be talked through the various options so that you can decide which you feel is likely to work best for you. You will be offered regular follow-up appointments to monitor your progress and support you as you quit. I know it can seem a hassle to have to attend appointments if you have a busy schedule, but these appointments are well worth prioritising as they will help you succeed.

DR DAWN'S TOP TIP

Spend some time thinking about why and when you smoke, so that you can identify your weak moments. For many, it will be with a drink at the end of a busy day, so perhaps planning to join friends who don't smoke, or making sure that you have your nicotine replacement at hand, will help you not to give in to those weaknesses. There will be other less obvious triggers, and knowing what they are for you will mean you are less likely to succumb.

HOW DO I COPE WITH CRAVINGS?

Cravings are, I'm afraid, an inevitable part of giving up, but they're not insurmountable. If cravings are a problem for you, then you may be a good candidate for one of the targeted medications. It is also important that you formulate a plan to deal with the cravings – as bad as they are, they don't last forever. One lovely patient of mine dealt with her cravings by having a shower every time they got too intense. It took me a while to understand her logic, but it was very simple – she couldn't smoke in a shower, so by the time she was out of the shower, she had found her willpower. That was a perfect solution for her as she worked from home. It isn't practical if you are based in an office, but there will be something you can plan to do when the going gets tough to distract you long enough to find the willpower to carry on.

DR DAWN'S TOP TIP

Plan ahead. By setting a quit date, you can make sure that you have got rid of all your cigarettes (if that is part of your plan). And go public! Telling everyone what you are doing will help your motivation and means your friends and family can support you. Put aside the money you would spend on cigarettes each week for something special, as your reward, or add it to a sponsorship fund and raise money for a charity that your supporters can donate to.

HOW SOON WILL I REAP THE BENEFITS OF GIVING UP SMOKING?

This is where the good news starts – the health benefits of giving up smoking start straight away. Check this out – after:

- 20 minutes, your pulse rate starts to return to normal
- 8 hours, oxygen levels return to normal and carbon monoxide levels in your blood reduce by more than 50%

- 48 hours, you will no longer have carbon monoxide in your blood and your lungs will start to clear out mucus and other debris
- 72 hours, your airways will begin to relax, meaning your breathing gets easier and you should start to feel more energised
- 2–12 weeks – this is where things start to change for your long-term health. During this period, if you have managed to stay off cigarettes, your circulation will generally improve
- 3–9 months, you can expect your lung function to have improved by as much as 10%
- 1 year – this is a real milestone! If you have given up for a year, your risk of heart disease is half that of a smoker
- 10 years – remember all those horrid statistics about lung cancer? If you have given up for 10 years, your risks of lung cancer are half what they were!
- 15 years, your risk of heart disease is now that of a non-smoker. I know smokers (quite rightly) often describe themselves, even years after successfully giving up, as a 'smoker who hasn't had a cigarette in x years', but now you are, in terms of your health, a non-smoker!

ALCOHOL

It is estimated that nine million people in the UK are regularly drinking over the recommended limits, which is likely to be a significant underestimate, as we rely on individual reporting of alcohol consumption to assess this. Most people (intentionally and unintentionally) underestimate their consumption – but more of that later. It's a serious problem because each year, approximately 9,000 people in the UK die of alcohol-related deaths, and health statisticians tell us that alcohol accounts for 10% of the UK burden

of disease and death. That makes alcohol the third lifestyle risk factor
for disease and death, after obesity and smoking. The bottom line is
that alcohol costs the NHS £3.5 billion per year – that's £120 per
year, per taxpayer.

WHAT HAS HAPPENED TO DRINKING IN THE UK?

When I was a child, my mother would often have a gin and tonic as
she was preparing supper, but I don't remember wine being in the
house, unless she was entertaining. Today, we are much more likely
to drink wine with a meal in the home. I also remember sipping
cider at parties in my teens, whereas today, young people are opting
for alcopops and spirits as their drinks of choice. Drinking behaviour
has changed in the UK.

And this is borne out by the statistics. Today, only 18% of
British adults say they don't drink at all, and 17% of men and 12%
of women admit to regularly drinking above recommended limits,
with 5% of men and 4% of women reporting heavy alcohol
consumption of greater than 50 and 35 units per week
respectively.

WHAT ARE CURRENT RECOMMENDED LIMITS?

Current guidelines from the Chief Medical Officer state that both
men and women should drink no more than 14 units of alcohol in
any week. These guidelines came into place in 2016 and are tougher
than previous guidelines, which allowed men 21 units a week, and
women 14. The change came after years of work looking at the
health effects of alcohol and, as evidence has come to light about
the link between alcohol consumption and serious health problems
(including liver disease, heart disease and several cancers), advisors

are telling us that we need to be even more careful about our intake.

Guidelines for pregnant women have also changed. We used to say that it was OK to have one or two units once or twice a week, but now recommendations are to abstain completely from alcohol while pregnant. This isn't because we have any new evidence that those low levels cause lasting damage, but because we know that alcohol isn't going to do an unborn baby any good, so total abstinence is preferable.

One thing is for sure – if you want to live a long and fulfilled life, watching your alcohol intake is a priority!

WHAT IS A UNIT?

We used to say that a unit was a small glass of wine, a single measure of spirit or half a pint of beer. The problem is, beers and wines have become stronger over the years, so a home-poured glass of wine could be more than three units – this is what I mean about unintentionally underestimating your alcohol intake. If you pour a couple of glasses of wine in an evening, you might innocently tell your GP that you drink 14 units a week (7 × 2) whereas in fact you are probably drinking nearer 42 (7 × 6), and you are also omitting any extra that you might drink at the weekend. If you want to calculate your units accurately, there is a simple formula you can use. Look at the percentage of the alcohol you are drinking. To make the maths easy, let's say you drink 12% wine (most wines today are stronger than this). The percentage of alcohol is equivalent to the number of units in a litre of that fluid. This means that 12% wine has 12 units in a litre and that means three-quarters of twelve in a 75-centilitre standard-sized bottle; in other words, nine units in a bottle. If you are drinking large (250 ml) glasses, then a glass of wine is three units, not one.

DR DAWN'S TOP TIP

Next time you put out your recycling, give yourself some time to look at the percentage of alcohol on the bottles and calculate your household intake. Even excluding what you may have drunk away from home, you are likely to be surprised! This may help you cut down, especially if you start to look at the number of calories that equates to . . .

ALCOHOL AND CALORIES

Get ready to be scared! Calories in alcohol (see Table 3.1) are what we call empty calories, in that they have no nutritional value. Also, alcohol plays havoc with your willpower. When drinking alcohol, you are more likely to snack on crisps, nuts and canapés, which are loaded with extra calories.

Table 3.1: The calories in alcohol.

Alcohol	%	Size	Units	Calories
Wine	14	125 ml glass	1.8	105
Champagne	12	125 ml glass	1.5	95
Cider	7.5	500 ml can	3.8	230
Beer	5	330 ml bottle	1.7	134
Beer	4	pint	2.3	180
Alcopop	4	275 ml bottle	1.1	164
Dark spirit	40	25 ml single	1.0	61
White spirit	37.5	25 ml single	0.9	52

WHAT IS A BINGE?

I'm sure most of you would not describe yourselves as binge drinkers. Bingeing is the sort of behaviour you see outside a nightclub on a Saturday night, with people staggering all over the place, vomiting on the pavement and falling over, isn't it? Sorry, no!

The definition of a binge used by the Office of National Statistics is more than eight units in one session for a man, and more than six for a woman. Go back to my calculations of a large home-poured glass of wine and suddenly you will see how easy it is to binge – if a woman has more than a couple of large glasses of wine in one evening, she is bingeing!

The problem with binge drinking is that, as a rough guide, your liver can process about one unit of alcohol per hour. This varies from person to person – people who drink regularly may process alcohol more quickly – but, if you are drinking several units in a short time, this will put extra strain on your liver, as well as clouding your judgement and making you more prone to accidents. Remember, we are aiming for a long and healthy life – an accident following a silly mistake could increase your risk of developing serious problems later in life and curtail your quality of life.

DR DAWN'S TOP TIP

Avoid bingeing by getting into the habit of alternating alcoholic drinks with soft drinks. This will keep you well hydrated (alcohol is a diuretic and some hangover symptoms are caused by dehydration) and will cut your unit consumption by half on a night out.

ALCOHOL AND DRIVING

I am often asked how much it is safe to drink before getting behind the wheel. The honest answer to that is: nothing. We absorb and process alcohol at different rates, and the same person will vary in how they handle alcohol from day to day – for example, if you have had a big meal, you will absorb alcohol more slowly than if you are drinking on an empty stomach. The legal alcohol limit for driving in England, Wales and Northern Ireland is 80 mg of alcohol for every 100 ml of blood in your body, or 35 mg of alcohol for every 100 ml of breath. In Scotland, it is less – 50 mg of alcohol per 100 ml of blood, or 22 mg of alcohol per 100 ml of breath, which is in line with most other European countries. These aren't arbitrary levels. Even a small amount of alcohol in your blood can affect your reaction times and judgement. Each year, approximately 250 people die in accidents in which at least one driver was over the drink-drive limit. Patients of mine have lost loved ones in such an accident – or been the drunk driver. Of the people I know who have been drunk when driving, they aren't bad or irresponsible people by nature. They would never describe themselves as drink drivers, but they made a mistake and paid a huge price for it. Living a long and healthy life is not just about physical health; it's also about good mental health, and feeling remorseful for causing an accident such as this could lead to years of recrimination and guilt.

DR DAWN'S TOP TIP

Offer to drive when you go out – it gives you the perfect excuse not to drink. It is easy to feel pressurised into drinking, but if you're driving, people will not offer you drinks.

ALCOHOL AND THE LIVER

The liver is the second largest organ in our body (skin is the largest) and it does over 500 different jobs, including breaking down our food, getting rid of waste products, helping fight infection, and making sure our blood clots appropriately. When it fails, we die – plain and simple. The worrying thing is that when your liver is under strain, you may have no warning signs whatsoever. People expect that they will become jaundiced (a condition in which the liver struggles to work properly, which in turn allows bilirubin levels to rise, leading to a yellow tinge to the whites of the eyes and skin) or develop abdominal pain, but your liver can be in quite a bad way and you may have no idea.

The liver sees alcohol as a poison, and works hard to clear it from your system. When alcohol is broken down, the resulting chemical reaction can damage the liver cells. The amazing thing about the liver is that it has incredible powers of regeneration. The first stages of damage will be a fatty infiltration of the liver – this also happens in overweight people. If this is picked up, and you stop drinking, the liver will repair itself; if you carry on drinking, you risk developing inflammation in the liver (alcoholic hepatitis). This may have no symptoms and, even at this point, if you stop drinking, the liver can recover. However, if this goes unnoticed (which it easily can), and you continue to drink, you risk developing cirrhosis. Cirrhosis is irreversible and increases the risk of liver cancer. Liver disease is the only major cause of death increasing in the UK – twice as many people die from liver disease in the UK today than 25 years ago. More than 16,000 people will die in this country this year from liver disease, and alcohol is by far the leading cause. You don't want to be one of them.

DR DAWN'S TOP TIP

Don't wait for warning signs. They may not come. Your liver can't tell you if you are drinking too much, but you can. Be honest with yourself about your consumption and, if you are drinking too much, start by putting a couple of dry days in your diary. A lot of over-drinking is habit rather than addiction: look at ways of changing your habits. If you feel you have a more serious problem, don't ignore it – speak to your GP.

ALCOHOL AND CANCER

One in three of us will develop cancer in our lifetime, and I will talk more about how we can reduce our risks in Chapter 8, but let me give you one hard-and-fast fact now – the less alcohol you drink, the lower your risks of developing cancer. Don't get me wrong – I'm not suggesting we should all become teetotal. I love a glass of wine and will be the first to admit that I don't always stick to recommended limits: for example, this year I had a 'dry' January because I know I had a rather 'wet' December! It's all about balance. I appreciate that we live in a society where it is all too easy to drink more than we should, but we mustn't lose sight of the real health risks (if we don't rein ourselves in). They include some serious diseases:

- **head and neck cancer – people who regularly drink more than 3.5 drinks a day have a two- to three-fold increased risk of developing these cancers, and if you smoke as well, the risks are significantly higher**
- **oesophageal cancer**
- **liver cancer**
- **breast cancer – women who drink three drinks a day have a 1.5 times higher risk of developing breast cancer than non-drinkers, and the risk continues to rise with every extra drink per day**
- **bowel cancer – drinking 3.5 drinks a day increases the risk of bowel cancer by 1.5 times.**

Researchers have identified several ways in which alcohol increases the risk of developing cancer, and it seems to be related to the toxic effects of the breakdown products of alcohol, which can damage DNA and proteins, allowing the cancers to begin.

CAN RED WINE HELP PREVENT CANCER?

Much has been written about the possible health benefits of drinking red wine – and there are some. The theory behind red wine having a protective effect against cancer is that it contains a substance called resveratrol, which is known to have anti-cancer properties. It is also found in grapes, raspberries and peanuts. But, despite lots of research, any protective effect is yet to be proven. I suspect that is because, to consume the required amounts of resveratrol, we would have to drink so much red wine that any benefit would be far outweighed by its detrimental effects – sorry!

ALCOHOL AND HEART DISEASE

Alcohol can affect the heart in many ways. Consistently over-drinking will raise blood pressure, putting a strain on the heart. It is also likely to lead to weight gain, which will add to the problem. Excess drinking can also affect the way the heart muscle pumps, making it weaker and less effective, and binge drinking can trigger an abnormal heart rhythm.

The good news is that drinking within recommended limits can be good for your heart – alcohol raises good cholesterol known as high density lipoproteins (HDLs) and makes you less prone to clots. But don't use this as an excuse to pour an extra glass – the beneficial effects are only for moderate drinking, and the risks of heavy drinking far outweigh any benefits.

DR DAWN'S TOP TIP

If you know you are regularly drinking more than you should, get your blood pressure checked. Contrary to popular belief, most people with high blood pressure don't have headaches or problems with their vision. If you don't get it checked you won't know if there are any problems, and if it is high, maybe it will be the warning you need to get yourself back on track.

HOW DO I CUT DOWN ON MY DRINKING?

I've given you plenty of reasons to want to regulate your alcohol intake, but it isn't always that easy. Alcohol is readily available in our society and inherently linked to social situations and meeting up with friends. However, giving up or cutting down is not impossible, and the health benefits you will reap are well worth the effort. Even a few alcohol-free days per week should leave you feeling more energised and sleeping better. People often use alcohol to help them get to sleep, and it is very effective for this, but what most people don't realise is that alcohol disrupts our normal sleep rhythms – while you may go to sleep more easily, you won't have the same quality of sleep, meaning that you wake the next day feeling less refreshed.

DR DAWN'S TOP TIPS

If you are looking to cut down on alcohol, here are a few simple things you can do that will help:

- Tell those closest to you – they will be able to encourage you in your weak moments and won't try to tempt you off-track.
- Alternate alcoholic drinks with soft drinks.
- Schedule two 'dry' days each week.
- Only allow yourself an alcoholic drink while you are eating your meal in the evening.
- Never pour yourself a drink – always wait to be offered. Topping up your glass can increase those units.
- Consider changing your choice of alcohol – if you know you drink wine like squash, for example, think about changing to a gin and tonic, which you may drink more slowly.
- Don't buy alcohol with your weekly shop. Supermarkets and off-licences are open all hours, but you will be less likely to reach for the bottle if it involves having to go out to get it!
- Try to get the people you live with to buy into the same philosophy. That way you will be able to encourage each other.

- Put aside the money you would have spent on alcohol and treat yourself to a reward.
- Recognise your triggers – if reaching for the wine bottle as soon as the kids are in bed has become a habit, think about what you will do instead, so that you are preoccupied and not tempted.

WHAT IF YOU ARE CONCERNED ABOUT SOMEONE ELSE'S DRINKING?

I am often asked for help by patients who are worried, not for themselves, but for people they love who they feel are drinking too much. This is a difficult one, because no one else can cut down or cut out alcohol for you. The chances are that the person has secret worries about their alcohol intake themselves, but it is vital that you pick the right moment. Never challenge anyone on their long-term drinking habits when they have already had a few drinks. This is a conversation for the sober light of day. Try to be open, sensitive and empathic. Accusations and using words like 'alcoholic' are unlikely to be helpful. It's also a good idea to have some practical suggestions to hand so that if your conversation goes the way you want, you have something positive to offer. That could be anything from cutting down together, planning what you will do with the saved money as a treat, or, for more serious problems, websites and self-help numbers. Remember, there's plenty of help available for people for whom drinking is a problem. If you are seriously worried about your drinking, your GP will be able to advise you on local services – you won't be the first and you certainly won't be the last, but you do need to get yourself back on track if you are going to give yourself the best chance of living a long and healthy life.

CHAPTER 4

DIABETES – A TWENTY-FIRST-CENTURY EPIDEMIC

I f I had been writing this book a few decades ago, I may not even have included this chapter, but the sad truth is that in the UK today, diabetes (or, to be more precise, type 2 diabetes) is one of the most significant factors affecting our longevity. It is estimated that there are 3.2 million people in the UK today with diabetes, 90% of them with type 2.

It is important that I differentiate between type 1 and 2 diabetes here. They really are very different diseases – so much so that I almost wish they had totally different names. I will briefly explain the differences below, and the rest of this chapter will refer to type 2 diabetes.

TYPE 1 DIABETES

Type 1 diabetes is an autoimmune disease, in which the human body recognises a part of its own being as foreign and develops antibodies to fight it. In type 1 diabetes the body fights against its pancreas, rendering it incapable of producing the essential hormone insulin. Insulin is needed to regulate blood sugar levels. Without it, glucose levels rise in the bloodstream.

In type 1 diabetes this results in excessive thirst (polydipsia) and the production of increasing amounts of urine (polyuria). It may also make the individual more prone to infection, and cause unexplained weight loss and abdominal pain. If left untreated, sugar levels continue to rise, leading to confusion and ultimately even convulsions, coma and death. If an individual develops type 1 diabetes, they will require insulin replacement therapy for life.

TYPE 2 DIABETES

Type 2 diabetes is usually, but not always, related to weight gain. In fact, when I was a medical student we were taught that type 1 diabetes was also called juvenile onset diabetes as it tends to occur in children and adolescents, while type 2 diabetes was referred to as maturity onset diabetes because it usually develops in mid-life, at a time when we tend to gain weight – specifically around our midriff. We are more politically correct today and the term 'middle-aged spread' is rarely heard. But just because we don't hear much about it doesn't mean it doesn't exist. It does! We all know people who seem to be able to eat what they like and stay irritatingly slim but for most of us, middle age is likely to bring a few extra pounds as our metabolism changes and that weight is usually deposited around our middles.

The terms 'juvenile onset' and 'maturity onset' were dropped at the start of the twenty-first century as we started to see children develop type 2 diabetes. The youngest person I have heard of being diagnosed with type 2 diabetes was a three-year-old child in America who was already classified as being morbidly obese.

Unlike type 1 diabetes, type 2 diabetes develops slowly. If it is picked up early it can often be managed with diet and lifestyle changes alone, but if left untreated patients often need prescription medication. Some people with type 2 diabetes may need insulin by injection.

Type 2 diabetes develops either because you have become resistant to the effect of insulin, so normal insulin levels aren't enough to keep your blood sugar under control, or because your body doesn't make enough insulin. In some cases it can be a mixture of the two.

Unlike type 1 diabetes, it is possible to have the condition but have no symptoms whatsoever. In fact, it is estimated that around 630,000 people in the UK have type 2 diabetes and don't yet know they do. If you are carrying excess weight – particularly around your middle – you could be one of them.

Diabetes, whether it is type 1 or 2, makes you prone to higher than normal sugar levels, and long-term high blood sugar damages nerves and blood vessels, causing heart disease, kidney disease, visual problems and peripheral vascular disease. I will come back to this later in this chapter.

DR DAWN'S TOP TIP

If you are at risk of type 2 diabetes (see below) don't wait for symptoms – make an appointment to see your GP or practice nurse for a check-up. An early diagnosis has a much better outlook. Currently a person diagnosed with type 2 diabetes has a 50% chance of already having complications of the disease, such as heart disease, kidney disease and an increased risk of stroke or blindness. Making the diagnosis earlier means you could avoid these debilitating conditions and live your life to the full for longer.

WHERE DOES BLOOD SUGAR COME FROM?

Blood sugar, also called blood glucose, comes from the food we eat. There are naturally occurring sugars in fruit (fructose) and milk (lactose) and obvious sources of sugar in, for example, cakes, biscuits and sweets. But if you start looking at food labels you will notice that you consume a lot more sugar than you might at first think. Processed foods and pre-packaged meals and sauces are often high in sugar. And healthy 'low-fat' products may not be as healthy as you think, as the fat is often replaced by sugar to enhance the taste.

Current recommendations are that adults should consume no more than 5% of their total daily calories in the form of free sugars. These include the sugar you add to food and drink as well as the sugar found naturally in honey, syrups, fruit juices and fruit juice concentrates. In real terms this means the average adult should consume no more than seven teaspoons (or 30 grams) of sugar a day. Given that a 330 ml can of fizzy drink contains around nine teaspoons (or 35 g) of sugar, it is easy to see why so many of us are consuming way above current recommendations.

Reading labels can be time consuming at first – but once you get into the habit of doing so, it can be very revealing. Many manufacturers now use a 'traffic light' labelling system – if you don't want to have to read every label, sticking to green or amber products wherever possible and limiting red products to occasional treats is a good way to start.

DR DAWN'S TOP TIP

Start looking at food labels so you can count the hidden sugars in your diet. Remember, you should be eating no more than 30 g of sugar a day. And if you can't be bothered with numbers, at least limit the red label products to high days and holidays. You will be surprised by how much 'hidden' sugar there is in your food. One can of cola, for example, could contain more sugar than your daily allowance. Spending a few minutes reading labels during your weekly shop could pay huge dividends in living well in later life.

APPLES AND PEARS

If I were to take twins of identical height and weight but one carried their weight around their middle (the classical apple shape) while the other carried their weight on their hips and thighs (the pear shape), then even though they may have the same body mass index (BMI), the apple-shaped twin would have a higher risk of heart disease, stroke and type 2 diabetes than the pear-shaped twin. This is because weight around the middle and around our internal organs is regarded as 'active fat'.

I think of it in terms of factories and warehouses. Weight on the hips and thighs is like a warehouse storing up fat to be used when supplies are needed, while fat on the waistline is like a factory actively producing hormones that increase the risk of disease. This is one of the reasons doctors are increasingly using waist circumference as a marker for disease.

To measure your waist, you need to feel for your hip bone and for the bottom of your ribs. Breathe out naturally (don't force your abdomen out, just gently exhale) and measure your circumference midway between these two points. It is a good idea to check the measurement more than once to ensure you have done this accurately – and no cheating! I have met hundreds of people happily walking around in 34-inch waist trousers which fit beautifully *below* their 44-inch waist.

Women should have a waistline no greater than 80 cm (31.5 inches) and men no greater than 94 cm (37 inches). Waistlines larger than this are associated with an increased risk of high blood pressure, heart disease and diabetes. If you are of Asian descent, things get even tougher. Asian men in particular are at increased risk of heart disease and type 2 diabetes, so your waistline should be no more than 90 cm (35.5 inches). Women with a waist greater than 88 cm (35 inches) and men with a waist greater than 102 cm (40 inches) are at high risk. If that is you, it is time to take yourself in hand and change your future by making some lifestyle changes to get your weight under control.

Doctors also sometimes use a measurement called the waist-to-hip ratio. To calculate this you measure your waist as described opposite – at the midpoint between your hip bone and the bottom of your ribs. Take your hip measurement at the widest point of your hips and calculate the ratio by dividing the waist number by the hip number. A ratio of 1.0 or more in men or 0.85 or more in women means you are carrying too much weight around your middle.

HOW MUCH FAT IS HEALTHY?

We need some fat to keep us insulated, to protect our organs, and as a source of stored energy. But excess fat is bad for us and increases our risk of heart disease, type 2 diabetes and high blood pressure – to name just a few. How much fat is healthy depends on your gender and age. Some scales will calculate your percentage of body fat for you, but you can do this yourself using the calculations below, an ordinary set of weighing scales, and a tape measure.

WOMEN

Body fat percentage = (1.20 × BMI) + (0.23 × age) – 5.4

MEN

Body fat percentage = (1.20 × BMI) + (0.23 × age) – 16.2

The following guidelines will help you work out whether you have anything to worry about.

WOMEN

AGED 20–40

- <21% = underweight
- 21–33% = healthy
- 33–39% = overweight
- >39% = obese

AGED 41–60

- <23% = underweight
- 23–35% = healthy
- 35–40% = overweight
- >40% = obese

AGED 61–79

- <24% = underweight
- 24–36% = healthy
- 36–42% = overweight
- >42% = obese

MEN

AGED 20–40

- <8% = underweight
- 8–19% = healthy
- 19–25% = overweight
- >25% = obese

AGED 41–60

- <11% = underweight
- 11–22% = healthy
- 22–27% = overweight
- >27% = obese

AGED 61–79

- <13% = underweight
- 13–25% = healthy
- 25–30% = overweight
- >30% = obese

DR DAWN'S TOP TIP

Calculate your percentage of body fat today using scales and a tape measure and look at the charts above. If you are overweight or obese, start thinking about small changes you could make to your lifestyle. This book lists all the changes you can make to change your future. It's never too late to start. Remember, you can have type 2 diabetes for years without having any symptoms.

WHAT ABOUT BODY MASS INDEX?

Body mass index (BMI) is also a good indicator of whether you are a healthy weight for your height. There are some exceptions to this, such as if you are very fit and muscly. Some top-level rugby players, for example, will be very fit but, because muscle is denser than fat, their BMI may put them in the overweight, or even obese, category. Since most of us are not top-flight rugby players, BMI still has a role to play.

To calculate your BMI you simply need to know your weight in kilos and your height in metres. Your BMI is your weight in kilos divided by the square of your height in metres:

$$BMI = \text{weight in kg}/(\text{height in metres})^2$$

Table 4.1: The BMI chart.

Weight (lbs)	100	105	110	115	120	125	130	135	140	145	150	155	160	165	170	175	180	185	190	195	200	205	210	215
Weight (kgs)	45.5	47.7	50.0	52.3	54.5	56.8	59.1	61.4	63.6	65.9	68.2	70.5	72.7	75.0	77.3	79.5	81.8	84.1	86.4	88.6	90.9	93.2	95.5	97.7
Category		UNDERWEIGHT				HEALTHY					OVERWEIGHT					OBESE					EXTREMELY OBESE			

Height (in / cm)	100	105	110	115	120	125	130	135	140	145	150	155	160	165	170	175	180	185	190	195	200	205	210	215
5'0" / 152.4	19	20	21	22	23	24	25	26	27	28	29	30	31	32	33	34	35	36	37	38	39	40	41	42
5'1" / 154.9	18	19	20	21	22	23	24	25	26	27	28	29	30	31	32	33	34	35	36	36	37	38	39	40
5'2" / 157.4	18	19	20	21	21	22	23	24	25	26	27	28	29	30	31	32	33	33	34	35	36	37	38	39
5'3" / 160.0	17	18	19	20	21	22	23	23	24	25	26	27	28	29	30	31	31	32	33	34	35	36	37	38
5'4" / 162.5	17	18	18	19	20	21	22	23	24	24	25	26	27	28	29	30	30	31	32	33	34	35	36	37
5'5" / 165.1	16	17	18	19	19	20	21	22	23	24	25	25	26	27	28	29	30	30	31	32	33	34	35	35
5'6" / 167.6	16	16	17	18	19	20	21	21	22	23	24	25	25	26	27	28	29	29	30	31	32	33	34	34
5'7" / 170.1	15	16	17	18	18	19	20	21	21	22	23	24	25	25	26	27	28	29	29	30	31	32	33	33
5'8" / 172.7	15	15	16	17	18	19	19	20	21	22	22	23	24	25	25	26	27	28	28	29	30	31	32	32
5'9" / 175.2	14	15	16	17	17	18	19	20	20	21	22	22	23	24	25	25	26	27	28	28	29	30	31	31
5'10" / 177.8	14	15	15	16	17	17	18	19	20	20	21	22	22	23	24	25	25	26	27	28	28	29	30	30
5'11" / 180.3	14	14	15	16	16	17	18	18	19	20	20	21	22	23	23	24	25	25	26	27	27	28	29	30
6'0" / 182.8	13	14	14	15	16	17	17	18	19	19	20	21	21	22	23	23	24	25	25	26	27	27	28	29
6'1" / 185.4	13	13	14	15	15	16	17	17	18	19	19	20	21	21	22	23	23	24	25	25	26	27	27	28
6'2" / 187.9	12	13	14	14	15	16	16	17	18	18	19	19	20	21	21	22	23	23	24	25	25	26	27	27
6'3" / 190.5	12	13	13	14	15	15	16	16	17	18	18	19	20	20	21	21	22	23	23	24	25	25	26	26
6'4" / 193.0	12	12	13	14	14	15	15	16	17	17	18	18	19	20	20	21	21	22	23	23	24	25	25	26

Alternatively, you can work it out using the chart shown in Table 4.1. A healthy BMI is between 18.5 and 25. A BMI over 25 is classed as being overweight and a BMI of over 30 is clinically obese. A BMI over 40 is deemed morbidly obese and, as its name implies, has serious implications for health and life expectancy.

Last year I met Carl Thompson, 'Britain's fattest man'. At just 32 years old, he weighed 65 stone. You don't need a medical degree to know he wasn't going to make old bones without some serious intervention, but sadly it was too late. Carl died a few months later at the age of 33. He was one of an increasing number of people in the Western world with a BMI over 50 who are described as the 'super-obese'.

I suspect that, after our genetic make-up, our weight (which, it could be argued, is often linked to genetics) will be one of the most important factors relating to longevity in the UK today.

DR DAWN'S TOP TIP

We know if we are carrying extra weight, and it can be easy to ignore it and put off weighing ourselves – but now is the time to take your head out of the sand. Use the equation above to calculate your BMI. If it is over 25 (you know what I am going to say!), you need to start working on your weight. Not simply because you want to fit into your favourite pair of jeans (although if that helps motivate you, I'm all for it!), but because bringing your BMI back into a healthy range will add years to your life.

GENETICS AND OBESITY

This is a fascinating field and one that is developing rapidly. Scientists are discovering more and more genes linked to a predisposition to weight gain. A few years ago, I was tested for twelve of the most common genes known to be associated with obesity. I tested positive for eight of them. My BMI is currently 21 so that may (on the face of it) seem an unlikely result, but I wasn't surprised. I have always been aware that I seem to put on weight more easily than my friends. I went away with a girlfriend last winter for a sunshine break. We pretty much ate and drank the same all week. The only real difference between our lifestyles that fortnight was that I swam 2 kilometres (1.24 miles) each morning while she teased me that I was supposed to be relaxing. We are a similar build. When we came back, I had gained half a stone while her weight had remained stable.

There are two ways of dealing with this. I can grumble that it's just not fair (which it isn't!), but until we find a way of manipulating our genetic profile it won't do any good; I will still put on weight more easily than my friend. The alternative is that I accept the facts and continue to watch what I eat and exercise regularly in order to avoid becoming overweight. I have opted for the latter, but it's not always easy – I am human so I let myself go a little on high days and holidays and then have to make an effort to rein myself back in.

Genetic testing for genes linked to a predisposition to gain weight is not available on the NHS, but can be requested privately. It involves providing a sample of saliva, which is then analysed in a laboratory.

HOW BIG A PROBLEM IS OBESITY?

Obesity really is a massive problem in the Western world. Nearly two-thirds of adults in England are overweight, and one in four Brits is now obese. One in five children leaves primary school overweight, which is a real worry, as children entering secondary school overweight are more likely to remain overweight as adults. Obesity levels in the UK have more than trebled in the past 30 years, and if we continue the way we are more than half the population could be obese by 2050. Life expectancy has been improving for decades, but experts are now predicting that this trend to increasing longevity could be about to reverse. The reason? Obesity. Even if being overweight doesn't shorten our lives, you have a higher risk of developing several illnesses.

Carl Thompson clearly had an unhealthy relationship with food – and many of us have a complex relationship with food. In the Western world, we rarely eat from genuine hunger. We are more likely to eat because it's sociable, it's a meal time, or food is just available. We eat when we are sad; we eat when we are happy. For Carl, eating had become bound up with emotional issues. Sadly, he passed away before receiving the psychological help he clearly needed.

According to the United Nations Food and Agriculture Organization the UK is, I'm afraid, top of Europe's obesity league. The figures below (for obesity rates in adults in each country) make depressing reading:

- UK – 24.8%
- Ireland – 24.5%
- Spain – 24.1%
- Portugal – 21.6%
- Germany – 21.3%
- Belgium – 19.1%
- Austria – 18.3%
- Italy – 17.2%
- Sweden – 16.6%
- France – 15.6%.[1]

DR DAWN'S TOP TIP

If you think you have a genetic predisposition to gain weight, you probably have. The important thing is that this is here to stay (at least, for now). You can't change it – but that doesn't mean you have to give in to it. If you are prone to weight gain you need to accept that you will have to work harder than others to maintain a healthy weight. In the long run, it will be worth the extra effort.

SO WE'RE GETTING BIGGER. DOES IT REALLY MATTER?

Well, I'm afraid as a doctor I have to say it does. With so many of us now overweight, it can be easy to be lulled into a false sense of security. Not that long ago, if you wanted to buy clothes in over a size 20, you would have to shop in an 'outsize shop'. The constant subliminal message was that you were overweight and not a 'normal' size. I am concerned that you can now buy larger and larger sizes off the peg in high-street stores: the message is that it's 'OK' and 'normal' to be that size.

And it's not just adults I'm talking about here. When I was at school, there were very few fat children. Looking back, it must have been pretty miserable to always be the last to be picked for sports teams. Today, in many schools, so many children are overweight that it has become the norm. You may remember a famous photograph of children playing in the street during World War II, their shirts off. At the 2017 Childhood Obesity Summit, this image was discussed. Chief Medical Officer Dame Sally Davies said: 'What worries me is how we have started to normalise it. In my generation it was normal to see [children's] ribs on the beach. That was healthy. How have we lost this national understanding of what is healthy and what is unhealthy?'[2]

Recently, the photo was shown to members of the public, who were asked whether they thought the children looked healthy. The majority of people thought they were underweight. They were actually a healthy weight, but that shows how our view of weight has changed over recent decades. We have got used to people being overweight so that people of a normal weight look underweight. The same goes for me – I have got so used to seeing bigger people in my surgery that I am often surprised when I weigh and measure patients who I am concerned may be clinically overweight, only to find they are not just overweight, but actually obese.

DR DAWN'S TOP TIP

We put on weight gradually. It's easy to kid ourselves that we haven't gained much, but most of us have a pair of 'thin jeans' or an old piece of clothing that we know we wouldn't be able to fit into any more but that we can't quite throw out . . . 'just in case'. Go and find that item now and try it on. It won't make you feel great, I'm afraid, but it might shock you into realising you have put on more weight than you thought. Keep that item of clothing – and let today be the first day of your journey back to that size. It may be a long journey, but it will be worth it.

I am often told that it is much easier to gain weight than it is to lose it. That's not actually true. It is true that it is much easier to consistently overeat by a few hundred calories a day than it is to restrict daily calories by the same amount. You will have bad days – you are human! It may take you months to get back into your jeans, but it will be worth it. Here I will show you how.

WHY ARE WE GETTING BIGGER?

We are living in what I call an obesogenic society. Food – and often the wrong food – is generally readily available, and we are living increasingly sedentary lives.

When my children were small, I encouraged them to be as active as possible and we spent a lot of time outdoors. But even with that way of life, I know that the advent of computers, PlayStations and Xboxes meant that my kids spent a lot more time sitting in front of a screen and were less active than I was at the same age. I, for example, would have hopped on my bike and cycled to see a friend at the weekend while my children would sit in their room chatting on Facebook. We often take childhood habits into adult life. Current recommendations are that British adults should walk 10,000 steps a day and exercise for 30 minutes at least five times a week. By 'exercise', I mean doing something that makes you puff, and a staggering 80% of us are falling short of this goal.

Our working lives are also different to a few generations ago. A couple of years ago, I decided to practise what I preach and bought myself a pedometer. Since I know I have a genetic predisposition to weight gain, I have always tried to stay active and on my non-surgery days I would do well over the 10,000 steps I should be taking. On busy days in surgery, though, it was a very different story – by the end of the working day, I would often only have done 2,000 steps. I appreciate that if you have a desk-based job, achieving recommended activity levels can be a challenge.

I decided to make some small changes: for example, to walk to the waiting room to call my patients in rather than using an intercom system. It made a big impact on my activity, and is a habit I have kept; it feels more personal. Our jobs are all different but, if you struggle with your weight, just promising you will use the stairs rather than the lift at work, or getting off the bus a stop early and walking from there to your office could make a big difference to your health and longevity (see Chapter 6).

Generations ago we wouldn't have needed to make such deliberate decisions to stay active. Let's think for a moment about Victorian times. All mothers would have been very busy. There were no televisions, washing machines, tumble dryers or vacuum cleaners. There were no cars to do the school run. She would have walked her children to and from school. She probably burned around 4,000 calories a day simply doing the household chores.

Today we estimate that the average adult woman needs 2,000 calories a day, and the average man 2,500. However, it is all too easy to exceed that calorific intake. For example, cereal for breakfast, a sandwich for lunch and an evening meal of fish or meat (or vegetarian alternative) with vegetables and a portion of carbohydrate such as potato, pasta or rice adds up to 2,000 calories. It is easy to see how adding a couple of snacks and milky or fizzy drinks could easily rack up the calories and lead to weight gain – without the individual feeling particularly overindulgent.

We have become a nation of grazers, and some experts believe that people who graze underestimate their daily calorie intake by between 500 and 1,000 calories a day.

DR DAWN'S TOP TIP

Invest in a pedometer – and use it! You may be surprised at how inactive you are. Just as I found calling in my patients in person helped me to achieve my 10,000 steps, you will be able to make small changes to your everyday life that will make it easier for you to get to 10,000 steps each day without even thinking about it.

WHAT IS A PORTION?

Recently, I visited a friend in hospital. It happened to be at a meal time, when a plate of fish and chips with a side order of peas was delivered to his bedside. The size of the fish was modest, served with a handful of chips and a good serving spoon-sized portion of peas. Compare that to a single portion of fish and chips at your average takeaway, and it is easy to see that we have got used to huge portion sizes. I tried not to buy many takeaways when my children were growing up, but as an occasional treat we would have fish and chips as a family. The portions were so huge that two or three portions would feed five of us. If we are going to live long and healthy lives we need to seriously rethink portion size.

I will talk more in the next chapter about what constitutes a healthy diet but the amounts listed below are appropriate portion sizes:

- grains – 1 slice of bread, 1 cup of rice, pasta or cereal
- fruit and vegetables – a tennis ball of fruit or veg, ½ a cup of canned fruit, a cup of salad or cooked veg

- dairy – four matchbox-sized cubes of cheese, one small pot of yoghurt, a cup of milk
- meat and alternatives – 3 oz of meat, poultry or fish, two small eggs or one large egg, two tablespoons of peanut butter
- oils, spreads and dressings – 1 teaspoon of dressing, oil, butter or cream.

DR DAWN'S TOP TIP

Spend some time thinking about those sizes I mention above. We have got so used to overeating that they probably seem ridiculously small – but they are not! Invest in smaller plates and glasses, and put all your food on your plate at once. A smaller plate will look fuller, and you will almost certainly eat less as a result. That will lead to easy weight loss.

THE LINK BETWEEN TYPE 2 DIABETES AND OBESITY

Type 2 diabetes is most commonly associated with being overweight. Some people develop type 2 diabetes while they are a healthy weight, but for the vast majority of people the condition is directly linked to weight gain and obesity. Obesity probably accounts for 80–85% of the overall risk of developing type 2 diabetes.

I have noticed a definite change in the way people react to the diagnosis. When I qualified as a GP 20 years ago, it was relatively uncommon for me to make a diagnosis of type 2 diabetes, and when I did it was met with serious concern by my patients and their families. Fast forward to today, and type 2 diabetes is so common that everyone knows someone who has the disease. In fact, 1 in 17 UK adults has diabetes (worldwide the figure is 1 in 11). Because it is so common, there seems to be a degree of complacency about the diagnosis. There is almost a feeling that type 2 diabetes is a 'mild' form of the disease. It isn't. Doctors are making 400 new diagnoses of type 2 diabetes every day in the UK, and around half of those diagnosed will *already* have complications of the disease.

The thing is, if you look at your friend, relative or work colleague with type 2 diabetes, they may look slightly overweight but you may think that otherwise they look well. However, they could already be developing heart disease, eye disease, kidney disease or peripheral vascular disease. These are all serious conditions that significantly impair quality of life and reduce life expectancy. By the time an individual is diagnosed with type 2 diabetes, they have a 50% chance of already having developed some of these complications. The risks make for scary reading. If you have diabetes you have a:

- **200% increased risk of developing heart disease or a stroke**
- **25% increased risk of developing kidney disease**
- **50% increased risk of developing glaucoma**
- **300% increased risk of developing cataracts**
- **3,000% increased risk of needing an amputation.**

Diabetes is the leading cause of preventable sight loss in working-age people in the UK. You don't need me to tell you that losing your sight or losing a limb is going to have a very negative impact on your quality of life, but the NHS performs over 100 amputations every week on people with diabetes in the UK.

The NHS currently spends £1 million every single hour on managing diabetes – 80% of this is spent on treating the complications of diabetes. We all need to think about this. If doctors continue to make 400 new diagnoses each day (and some experts predict this rate may actually increase if people at risk of diabetes don't make some life changes), then there will be 5 million people with diabetes by 2025. That's 5 million people with a reduced life expectancy and a reduced healthy life expectancy – and, to be honest, an NHS with a similar prognosis.

THAT'S THE BAD NEWS – SO WHAT'S THE GOOD NEWS?

I don't believe that we have to accept that the NHS will become bankrupt under the weight (excuse the pun) of diabetes care. We have to be realistic, though. If we don't halt the inexorable rise in cases of type 2 diabetes, then we could lose the NHS within our lifetime.

However, we can all do our bit to change this. I believe I have a responsibility as an individual, as a mum, as a GP, as a broadcaster and as an author. Whatever hats you wear, think about what you could do to help yourself and those around you to aim for a healthy weight. I believe we have a real chance – and the responsibility – to change the future.

CHAPTER 5

GOOD DIETS, BAD DIETS

Over the years, I have said countless times that there is no such thing as a bad food, but there are plenty of bad diets! That may sound strange coming from a doctor but I really don't believe that cream cakes are the devil incarnate or that chocolate should be banned from shops. However, I do believe these foods should be occasional treats and even then eaten in sensible doses. They only cause real trouble when they become part of your everyday diet. When my children were small we used to have what I called a 'treats cupboard'. I never had a lot of biscuits or cakes in the house but when we did, this was where they lived. I remember catching my youngest sitting on the floor in front of said cupboard working his way through the contents one day and we had a conversation about the definition of a treat. I still laugh about it now.

Also, we are all human and we all have our weaknesses. If you love chocolate and I ask you to promise yourself you will never eat it again, however hard you try and however much you want to succeed, chocolate will become a 'forbidden fruit' and you will focus on it more and more until you finally give in and eat not just a few squares but the whole bar. Banning foods like that just doesn't work!

Today, food is readily available – and all too often it is the wrong sort of food. I think there are three fundamental problems with modern-day eating which predispose us to weight gain, high blood pressure, high cholesterol, heart disease, type 2 diabetes and a myriad of other conditions that threaten to cut our lives short and impact on our quality of life in later years.

These are quite simply:

• **processed foods**
• **snacks**
• **portion sizes.**

I will deal with all these in this chapter, but let's start by defining what we mean by a healthy, well-balanced diet.

WHAT IS A BALANCED DIET?

Eating a healthy, well-balanced diet will help to ensure we live well for decades to come, so let's look at the basic principles here. Our meals should be based on starchy foods and should include a wide variety of foods, including five portions of fruit and vegetable every day. Meals should also include some meat and fish (or alternatives for vegetarians and vegans), some fat, and dairy products. Recently, the British Medical Association has called for the government to recommend that we aim for ten portions of fruit and vegetables a day. For the moment, the government has decided that, given two-thirds of British adults eat under three portions per day, we should focus on trying to ensure people eat five for now. I believe that ten would certainly be healthier. I aim for two portions of fruit and at least five portions of vegetables each day. There is increasing evidence that plant-based eating is better for our health and longevity. You should try to include vegetables of all colours.[1]

STARCHY FOODS

Starchy foods should comprise about a third of our total daily food
intake. They are an excellent source of energy and include bread,
potatoes, cereals, rice, pasta and couscous. They are also a good
source of fibre, which is essential for bowel health. Many of us don't
eat enough fibre – current guidelines are that we should eat around
18 g of fibre each day. Starchy foods have, I think incorrectly, been
demonised in recent years, with fans of the Atkins diet blaming them
for weight gain. Starchy foods, if eaten in moderation, won't make
you gain weight. In fact, gram for gram, starchy foods contain less
than half the calories of fat. It's not the bread, potatoes and pasta
that will make you put on weight; it is more likely to be the butter,
oil and sauces you add to these foods.

Complex carbohydrates (like those found in wholegrains) are the
best for us as we digest these more slowly and therefore we feel
fuller for longer. Wholegrain varieties include wholemeal bread,
wholewheat pasta and brown rice.

FAT

We need some fat in our diet as a store of energy and also to
protect our vital organs from injury, but sadly most of us in the
Western world eat too much fat. This results in weight gain and high
cholesterol, which predisposes us to heart disease. If we want to live
a long and healthy life, we need to get serious about our fat intake.

Fat contains 9 calories per gram, compared to just 4 per gram for carbohydrates, sugar and protein, so it is easy to see how a high-fat diet can lead to weight gain. Fat should form no more than 35% of your total daily intake. Remember there are different types of fat, some of which are more harmful than others. Saturated fats and trans fats are the worst. Saturated fats are found in cakes, biscuits, butter, lard, cream, sour cream, crème fraiche, meat pies, sausages, the white fat on cuts of meat, coconut oil, coconut cream and palm oil.

People are often confused by trans fats, but the bottom line is that they are bad news and wherever possible they should be avoided, or at least kept to a minimum. Trans fats are formed when oil goes through a process called hydrogenation. Trans fats are sometimes also referred to as hydrogenated fats, so look out for that word on food labels too, and avoid it whenever you can. Processed foods, margarine, cakes and biscuits often contain trans fats. Trans fats can also occur naturally in some animal-based foods such as meat and dairy products.

Saturated and trans fats will raise your cholesterol, but unsaturated fats (like those found in vegetable oils such as rapeseed or olive oil and low-fat spreads) can actually help to lower your cholesterol.

If your budget will stretch to it, spreads fortified with plant stanols and sterols can help lower your cholesterol. Stanols and sterols occur naturally in small amounts in many grains, vegetables, fruits, legumes, nuts and seeds. Since they have powerful cholesterol-lowering properties, manufacturers have started adding them to foods (such as Flora Proactive and Benecol). Several of my patients have managed to avoid having to take statins by altering their diet and including these spreads. Statins are a family of drugs used to control cholesterol levels. Since only 20% of our cholesterol comes from our diet (the other 80% is made by our bodies, so that is back to genetics), statins are essential to control cholesterol. However, for many, a little manipulation of the diet may be all that is necessary

Natural sources of plant stanols and sterols include fruit, vegetables, nuts and seeds.

DR DAWN'S TOP TIP

Always remove any visible fat from cuts of meat before cooking, and use small amounts of vegetable oil or sunflower oil (rather than butter, margarine or ghee) when cooking.

HOW DO I KNOW IF I'M EATING TOO MUCH FAT?

Again, the answer is to pay attention to food labels when shopping. As a rough guide, more than 20 g per 100 g of fat is high in fat, and less than 3 g per 100 g is low, with anything in between being medium. Some labels will refer to 'saturates'. This means saturated fat, and more than 5 g of fat per 100 g is high, and less than 1.5 g is low, with anything in between being medium in fat.

ARE LOW-FAT OPTIONS THE BEST CHOICE?

We certainly need to watch our fat intake, but we should also be careful with low-fat foods. Fat is what makes our food tasty. In blind tastings, higher-fat varieties are consistently scored as being tastier than low-fat alternatives. If manufacturers are taking fat out of a food, they need to find a way of enhancing the flavour. They often do this by adding sugar, so check those labels.

DR DAWN'S TOP TIP

Public Health England has created an app that will read the barcodes of thousands of products and tell you instantly the fat, sugar and salt content of foods. It's called Food Smart – download it today. It will almost certainly alter the way you shop the next time you go to the supermarket!

SUGAR

Most of us are eating too much sugar. The government's most recent National Diet and Nutrition Survey[2] found that, overall, Brits are failing to eat enough fruit and veg, while our consumption of red meat and saturated fat is too high. But the most alarming discovery related to young children. Children aged between four and 10 drank 100 ml of sugary drinks per day on average in 2012/14 – a drop from 130 ml per day in 2008/10, the survey showed. But sugar still makes up 13% of children's daily calorie intake – nearly three times the 5% recommended limit.

Frighteningly, half of that sugar is eaten before the school day starts. The problem is, there is a lot of hidden sugar in our foods. It's not the sugar that we add to tea or coffee that is causing the real problem here (although it is best not to add sugar to drinks if you can); it's the sugar in packaged foods that really stacks up. The app I mentioned above will really help you here – and will probably shock you a bit too. The sugar content of foods is shown as lumps of sugar. Did you know that the average can of fizzy drink contains around 9 teaspoons of sugar?

Current recommendations are that adults should eat no more than 30 g per day of added sugar (that is sugar added to food by food manufacturers or ourselves, as opposed to naturally occurring sugars in fruit and dairy products). That is roughly 7 teaspoons of sugar. I believe that sugar should make up no more than 5% of your total daily calorie intake. The limits are lower for children – children aged four to six should have no more than 19 g (5 teaspoons of sugar) per day and seven- to ten-year-olds no more than 24 g (9 teaspoons of sugar). Remember what I said about the can of fizzy drink? Yes, that makes up a child's entire daily recommended sugar intake!

HOW DO I KNOW IF I AM EATING TOO MUCH SUGAR?

Look at the labels of the food you eat. You need to look for the 'carbohydrates (of which sugars)' figure. More than 20 g per 100 g is a high sugar content and less than 5 g per 100 g is low, with everything else in between being medium. Just like the fat content labels, some will be colour-coded. You should set yourself the same rules, aiming for mainly green products and restricting your red products to treats only.

There are limitations to this labelling, however, as the number shows you the total sugar and doesn't break it down into added sugars, which are the ones we need to cut down on, rather than sugars that are found naturally in fruit or milk, for example. Nevertheless, you can get an idea of the added sugar content by looking at the ingredients part of the label. The list always starts with the main ingredient first, so if sugar is up near the top you can assume you are looking at a high-sugar food. Remember – sugar may be listed under other names, including sucrose, glucose, maltose, fructose, corn syrup, honey, hydrolysed starch, invert sugar and molasses.

SUGAR AND YOUR TEETH

If you are eating sugary foods it is better to do this in one go rather than having several small portions throughout the day, as repeated exposure to sugar is more damaging to your teeth. We want to live well into old age and we want to look as good as we can too. There's nothing like rotten teeth to age you!

DR DAWN'S TOP TIP

Swap your breakfast fruit juice for a piece of whole fruit. Whole fruit has more nutrients than juice, and less sugar.

FRUIT AND VEGETABLES

I have already mentioned that we should be eating at least five portions of fruit and veg a day, but this doesn't necessarily have to be fresh fruit and veg. Frozen, canned and dried fruit and veg all count. It's important we try to achieve this, as several studies have shown that a high intake of fruit and vegetables reduces our risk of developing heart disease and some cancers. A portion is defined as 80 g. In real terms this is:

- 1 apple, banana, pear, orange, peach or similar-sized fruit
- 2 plums or apricots or similar-sized fruit
- 1 slice of melon or pineapple
- half a grapefruit or avocado
- 3 heaped tablespoons of fruit salad
- 1 heaped tablespoon of dried fruit
- 1 150 ml glass of juice
- 1 cupful of cherries or grapes
- 3 heaped tablespoons of vegetables
- 1 dessert bowl of salad.

Remember that potatoes, in this context, don't count as one of your five-a-day, because they are classified as a source of starch, but sweet potatoes, parsnips, turnips and swede do. Beans and pulses can also count as one portion, but no matter how much you eat of these they will only ever count as one portion: although they are an excellent source of fibre, they contain fewer nutrients than other fruit and veg.

Similarly, a 150 ml glass of fruit juice will count as one of your portions, but you can only count one glass as part of your five-a-day, because a lot of the fibre in fruit is lost during the juicing process.

FISH

We should be eating two portions of fish every week. This can be fresh, frozen, canned or smoked (but beware of the salt content in some canned or smoked fish). A portion is about 140 g and at least one of our fish portions should be oily fish as these are rich in omega 3 fatty acids, which protect against heart disease and reduce triglyceride levels. (Triglycerides are another form of fat in our bloodstream. Just like cholesterol, high levels increase the risk of heart disease.)

They have anti-inflammatory properties too, and it is thought that they may help to prevent arthritis. I have met far too many people over the years who have a perfectly active mind in later life but who can't live life to the full because of painful arthritis, so if you are aiming for an active retirement, you will need to stock up on your omega 3s – and keep doing so. We can't store omega 3s, so it is important that we keep up our dietary intake. Mackerel, sardines, pilchards, herring, sprats, whitebait, salmon, trout and fresh tuna are all oily fish. I'm sure it's no coincidence that all the centenarians I have met while researching this book have loved fish. If you really don't like fish, other dietary sources of omega 3s include flaxseed oil, fish oil, fish roe, seafood, chia seeds, walnuts, soybeans and spinach. Tinned tuna doesn't count, I'm afraid, because a lot of the omega 3 fatty acids are reduced during the canning process, so the omega 3 content of tinned tuna is similar to that of non-oily fish. (The same isn't true of sardines and pilchards because these fish are canned whole.)

DR DAWN'S TOP TIP

If you are not eating the recommended intake of oily fish, you should consider taking a supplement to protect your heart and joints for a healthy old age.

MEAT

Meat is a good source of protein, vitamins and minerals including iron, selenium, zinc and the B vitamins. It is one of the main sources of vitamin B12, which is only found naturally in animal-sourced foods such as meat and milk. Current recommendations are that eaters of red meat limit their intake to 70 g a day. That's an average – actually, it should be 88 g per day for men and 52 g per day for women. That's probably less than you think – an 8 oz steak equals 226 g! A cooked breakfast might include a couple of sausages and two rashers of bacon, which is likely to be almost twice the daily limit at 130 g. Four in ten men and one in ten women in the UK eat more than 90 g of red meat a day. It is likely that there is a link between eating red and processed meat and developing bowel cancer,[3] so you may want to cut back on these meats. Red meat includes beef, lamb, pork, veal, venison and goat. Duck, goose, game birds and rabbit do not count as red meat. Processed meat means the meat has been preserved by smoking, curing, salting or adding preservatives; examples include sausages, bacon, ham, salamis and pâté.

DR DAWN'S TOP TIP

Have at least one meat-free day per week to cut down on your total consumption of red meat.

MILK AND DAIRY

Milk and dairy products such as cheese and yoghurt are important sources of calcium and vitamin B, and should form part of a healthy, balanced diet. Calcium is vital for healthy bones. Our bones increase in density and strength up to our mid-twenties and then plateau before we start to lose density from our mid-thirties onwards. It is particularly important for women to eat enough calcium. Our bones are smaller and lighter than men's bones, so we have less to lose in the first place, and after the menopause our oestrogen levels drop, so we lose the protective effect oestrogen had on our skeleton, making us more prone to osteoporosis (sometimes known as brittle bone disease). Osteoporosis is totally painless until your bones become so brittle that they fracture if you fall. You will have seen little old ladies who are bent over and hunched. This is usually because the vertebrae in their spine have become so thin that they begin to crumple. These fractures are excruciatingly painful and have a dreadful impact on quality of life. Prevention is better than cure – and ensuring an adequate calcium intake is an important part of keeping osteoporosis at bay. Some people may have an allergy or intolerance to dairy foods: if this is you, make sure you speak to a dietician about how to maintain a good source of calcium in your diet. Being underweight is also a risk factor for osteoporosis, particularly in women, as very thin women have lower oestrogen levels.

EGGS

Eggs are an excellent source of protein. They also contain essential vitamins and minerals, including vitamins A, B2, B12 and D, folate and iodine. I am often asked about the cholesterol content of eggs. While they do contain cholesterol, the NHS has no recommended limit on the number of eggs you can eat each day. Today, as a result of changes in farming and feeding practices, British Standard eggs contain less cholesterol than they used to.

DR DAWN'S TOP TIP

Look for the red British Lion quality mark on eggs and egg boxes. This tells you that the eggs have been produced to the highest standards of food safety.

SALT

Too much salt will raise your blood pressure and put a strain on your kidneys, but how much is too much? Adults should aim to keep their salt intake to under 6 g per day. That is the equivalent to 2.4 g of sodium (which is how salt is sometimes recorded on food labels). Many people are surprised to hear that most of the salt we consume comes from bought food products, rather than from the salt we add to cooking or that we put on our plate when eating. A quick check of food labels will tell you how much salt there is in the food you are buying. Beware pre-packaged foods and sauces – they are often high in salt. As a guide, when you are looking at food labels, more than 1.5 g of salt per 100 g is high in salt, less than 0.3 g per 100 g is low, and anything in between has a medium level of salt.

DR DAWN'S TOP TIP

Try not adding salt to your food when cooking. It may taste a little bland at first, but you could add herbs and spices instead. You will be amazed by how quickly your taste buds acclimatise. After a couple of weeks you will wonder how you ever managed to eat such salty food!

VITAMINS, MINERALS AND TRACE ELEMENTS

Vitamins, minerals and trace elements are essential for a healthy life. This section looks at these individually, lists the foods that contain each of them, and says why we need them.

Vitamin A (also called retinol) – This vitamin is essential for eye health and in particular for helping us see in dim light. It is also necessary for healthy skin and to keep our immune system in good working order. It is found in milk and dairy products, eggs, oily fish and fortified spreads. It is present in high amounts in liver and liver-based products such as pâté. Beta-carotene (found in carrots, sweet potatoes, red peppers, spinach, apricots, mango and papaya) can be converted to vitamin A by the body, so these foods are also a good source. Men need an average of 0.7 mg a day and women 0.6 mg (there is around 0.5 mg in one carrot). If you consume more than this, your body will store the excess for future use. You should avoid eating liver or pâté more than once a week as there is some evidence that too much vitamin A could predispose you to osteoporosis.[4]

Vitamin B1 (also called thiamine) – This helps us break down and release energy from the food we eat. It is also needed to keep the nervous system healthy. It is found in fruit and vegetables, eggs, wholegrain bread, liver and some fortified cereals. Men need an average of 1 mg a day and women 0.8 mg (50 g of Brazil nuts contains 0.5 mg).

Vitamin B2 (also called riboflavin) – This helps us to release energy from our food, and plays a role in keeping our skin, eyes and nervous system in good shape. It is found in milk, eggs and rice as well as some fortified cereals. B2 is broken down by ultraviolet light, though, so it is important that these foods are stored out of direct sunlight to ensure that the vitamin content is not reduced. Men need an average of 1.3 mg per day and women 1.1 mg (there is around 0.75 mg in 100 g of rice).

Vitamin B3 (also called niacin) – This helps us release energy from food and keeps our skin and nervous system healthy. It is found in eggs, milk, meat, fish and wheat flour. Men need an average of 17 mg per day and women 13 mg (there is just over 20 mg in 100 g of cooked yellow tuna). In very high doses B3 can cause damage to the liver.

Vitamin B6 (also called pyridoxine) – This helps us use and store energy from protein and carbohydrates. It also makes haemoglobin (the protein in red blood cells that carries oxygen around the body). It is found in a wide variety of foods including pork, poultry, fish, eggs, bread, whole cereals, milk, vegetables, peanuts, potatoes and soya beans. Men need an average of 1.4 mg per day and women 1.2 mg (there is 0.8 mg in 100 g of chicken). Taking excessive doses of B6 (more than 200 mg a day) for a long time can affect the nerves in our arms and legs, resulting in altered sensation.

Vitamin B7 (also called biotin) – This is essential for the breakdown of dietary fat. It is found in a wide variety of foods but is also made by the bacteria in our gut, so our dietary intake is less important.

Vitamin B12 – This is used to make healthy red blood cells and to keep the nervous system healthy. It is found in animal products including meat, fish, eggs, milk and cheese. We need 2.4 mcg per day – a single serving of mackerel would give more than twice this amount.

DR DAWN'S TOP TIP

Water-soluble vitamins (vitamins B and C) can be destroyed by heat and they can be lost in water used for cooking. Wherever possible, steam or grill food to ensure the vitamin content is preserved.

Vitamin C (also called ascorbic acid) – This helps in wound healing. It is important for the health of connective tissues, which hold all our organs in place. People always associate oranges with vitamin C, but other good sources include strawberries, blackcurrants, red and green peppers, broccoli, sprouts and potatoes. Adults need 40 mg of vitamin C a day; there is 70 mg in an average orange. As it can't be stored, it should form part of your daily diet. Taken in excessive doses (>1000 mg), it can cause abdominal pain and diarrhoea.

Vitamin D – This regulates calcium and phosphate metabolism and is essential for healthy bones, teeth and muscles. Good sources include oily fish, red meat, liver and egg yolks. Some spreads and cereals are also fortified with vitamin D. This is an interesting vitamin because it needs sunlight for it to be activated. You only need to be out in the sun for 15 minutes a day, but in the UK between October and March, we don't get enough vitamin D from sunlight, so vitamin D deficiency is a common problem – so much so that doctors routinely recommend that breastfed babies aged under a year, children aged up to four, pregnant women and the elderly take a vitamin D supplement. Those who are housebound or who cover up their skin for religious or other reasons should also take a supplement.

Vitamin E – This is essential for healthy skin, eyes and the immune system. It is found in plant oils such as soya, corn and olive oil, nuts and seeds and wheat germ. Men need on average 4 mg per day and women 3 mg (there is 8 mg of vitamin E in 25 g of almonds).

Vitamin K – This helps blood to clot. It is found in green leafy vegetables, vegetable oils and cereal grains. Adults need 0.001 mg per kilogram of bodyweight per day – a cup of shredded raw green cabbage will give you more than half your daily requirement of vitamin K.

Boron – This is a trace element (meaning it is only present in minute amounts in a particular sample or environment). It helps the body use glucose, fat, calcium, copper and magnesium in our diet. It is found in green vegetables, fruit and nuts.

Calcium – There is more calcium in the body than any other mineral, and it's not just responsible for healthy bones and teeth; it also plays a vital role In the health and functioning of our muscles and in the clotting of blood. It is found in dairy products, green leafy vegetables, soya beans and drinks, tofu, nuts, pilchards and sardines. We need around 700 mg of calcium a day (although post-menopausal women may need more). If you eat too much calcium you may suffer from abdominal pain and diarrhoea. There is over 500 mg of calcium in one sardine.

Chromium – Another trace element. It helps insulin to regulate our blood sugar levels. It is found in wholegrains, lentils, spices, broccoli, potatoes and meat.

Cobalt – This is found in vitamin B12, so as long as you are getting B12 in your diet you will be getting cobalt. It is found in leafy green vegetables, nuts, cereals and fish.

Copper – You may not think of copper as a dietary element, but it is important for the production of red and white blood cells, and is also thought to play a pivotal role in brain development and in the maintenance of strong bones and a healthy immune system. It is found in nuts, shellfish and offal. Adults need 1.2 mg per day, and you should be able to get this from your normal diet. In high doses it can cause abdominal pain, sickness and diarrhoea.

Folic acid (also called folate) – This is essential for healthy red blood cells. All women planning a pregnancy and all pregnant women in the first trimester are advised to take a folic acid supplement, as it has been shown to reduce the risk of a foetus developing spina bifida. It is classified as one of the B-group vitamins. It is found in green vegetables such as sprouts, broccoli, peas, spinach and asparagus, and is also in liver and chickpeas. Men and women need 0.2 mg of folic acid a day (this equates to a cup of spinach). Since we can't store this vitamin, it is important that it forms part of our daily diet.

Iodine – This is needed to make thyroid hormones. It is found in sea fish and shellfish. It is also found in some grains, but levels will depend on the iodine in the soil in which they were grown. We need 0.14 mg a day (there is 0.3 mg in 100 g of saltwater fish).

Iron – This is important for the production of red blood cells. A lack of iron is a common cause of anaemia. It is found in dark green leafy vegetables, meat and liver, wholegrains, soybean flour, dried fruit and nuts. Men need 8.7 mg per day and women significantly more – 14.8 mg (because of blood loss from periods). There is 13 mg of iron in 100 g of chicken liver. High doses of iron can lead to constipation and abdominal pain.

Magnesium – This helps the parathyroid glands work well; these are essential for maintaining healthy bones. The parathyroid glands are four tiny glands (the size of a grain of rice) that sit in the neck and regulate calcium levels. Magnesium is found in fish, meat, dairy products, green leafy vegetables, nuts, brown rice and bread. Men need 300 mg a day and women 270 mg (there is 300 mg in a 100 g portion of fish). In high doses (more than 400 mg) it can cause diarrhoea.

Manganese – This is essential for healthy bones. It is found in tea, green vegetables, nuts, bead and cereals.

Molybdenum – This is probably the most important element – and you have probably never heard of it! It's essential for a healthy metabolism. The good news is, the daily recommended allowance is 45 micrograms (mcg). Most adults will get this from a balanced diet, so don't be tempted to take any supplements (unless advised to by a professional) as too much molybdenum is toxic. It is found in leafy vegetables, peas, cauliflower, nuts and cereals.

Nickel – This helps us absorb iron from our diet. It is found in lentils, oats and nuts.

Phosphorus – This is essential for healthy bones and teeth. It is found in meat, fish, dairy products, bread, brown rice and oats. Adults need 550 mg a day (there is 200 mg in a 100 mg portion of cod). Very high doses may cause abdominal pain and diarrhoea.

Potassium – This helps to balance fluids in the body and is needed to keep the heart muscle functioning properly. It is found in fish, shellfish, beef, poultry, Brussels sprouts, broccoli, parsnips, bananas, prunes, plums, pulses, nuts and seeds. Adults need 3,700 mg per day (there is over 400 mg of potassium in a banana, and 840 mg in a cup of spinach). Very high doses can cause abdominal pain, sickness and diarrhoea.

Selenium – This is needed for a healthy immune system and reproductive system. It is found in fish, meat, eggs and Brazil nuts. Men need an average of 60 mcg per day and women 50 mcg – there are 15 mcg in one egg. Too much selenium can cause thinning hair.

Silicon – This keeps bones and connective tissues healthy. It is found in fruit, vegetables and grains.

Sulphur – This helps your body make tissues, such as the cartilage found in joints. It is found naturally in all foods.

Zinc – This helps us to digest food, and also plays an important role in wound healing and making new cells. It is found in dairy products, meat, shellfish, bread and cereals. Men need 5.5–9.5 mg a day and women 4.0–7.0 mg (there is around 1 mg of zinc in a pitta bread). A high dose may inhibit the absorption of copper.

At first glance, this list may look quite daunting. However, if you look at the foods that provide each vitamin or mineral, there is a lot of overlap and you will probably be surprised at what you are managing to include in your diet. If you are concerned, keep an honest food diary for a couple of weeks (and I mean honest – if you cheat, you are only cheating yourself!) and ask a dietician to look over it. They will be able to tell you what, if anything, you need to change.

GENETICALLY MODIFIED FOODS – ARE THEY SAFE?

Arguments for and against GM foods have filled literally thousands of column inches in recent years, so what is the truth? Genetically modified foods are foods in which scientists have altered the genetic make-up of a food to enhance certain characteristics – taste, productivity, etc. Genetic modification has been happening for generations. No matter what you eat, it will be genetically different to the same food eaten by your ancestors. In nature, useful traits that help a plant or animal thrive will be passed on and eventually become more common. Human beings have been interfering with nature in this way for centuries by breeding from the best of a herd and saving the best of a crop to plant again for the next season. What genetic modification does is effectively fast-forward the whole process but, because of scientific advances, we can do that in a more targeted way. Genetic engineering has been used to enhance the vitamin content of some foods. However, it's not just about improving food quality; it is also about increasing quantity, or yield. Experts predict that some parts of the world will need to double their food production by 2050 to feed their expanding populations.

Many people have been concerned about the safety of GM foods, and the effects they may have on our health, but the World Health Organization (WHO) takes safety very seriously: the production of GM foods is tightly regulated and tested by top scientists so I am happy to include GM foods in my diet.

SHOULD I BE TAKING A SUPPLEMENT?

Certain people – such as post-menopausal women who don't have enough calcium in their diet, or elderly people in the UK who are at risk of vitamin D deficiency – should definitely take a supplement, and some of those I have mentioned during this chapter. Most of us should be able to get the nutrients we need from a well-balanced diet, but far too many of us don't achieve the government recommendations for all the food groups. If we are serious about improving our long-term health and longevity we need to look at ways of improving our diet – and, if necessary, supplementing it. Common nutrients that we may lack include vitamin B12 (especially in older people, who don't absorb as much B12 from their diet), calcium (especially post-menopausal women), vitamin D (the very young, the elderly, pregnant women, and those who are housebound or covered up), magnesium (it is often lost during processing, so may need to be supplemented), omega 3 fatty acids (if you're not a fish lover, you may not be getting enough of these and should consider supplementation).

If in doubt, have a chat with your doctor. As I read more about the body's ability to absorb vitamins and minerals past middle age, I have become more open to the idea of dietary supplementation, and have recently started taking a daily multivitamin.

HOW MUCH WATER SHOULD I DRINK EACH DAY?

The conventional answer to this question is eight glasses of water a day, but of course that depends on the size of your glasses! It also depends how much fluid you are getting from other sources, how warm it is, and how active you are, so I try not to get too hung up on actual quantities and simply tell my patients to look at their urine. Your urine should be straw-coloured – no darker. If it is darker than that then you need to drink more fluids – and don't wait until you feel thirsty to drink. Thirst is your body's reflex to dehydration, so you are already starting to become dehydrated by the time you are thirsty.

WHAT ABOUT PROBIOTICS?

I am a fan of probiotics. I take a daily probiotic and recommend them to a lot of my patients. Our guts are teeming with good bacteria that help us digest our food – we all have 2 kilos of bacteria living inside us, keeping our digestive system in balance. After suffering from diarrhoea, many of these bacteria are lost, which can prolong our symptoms as we don't have enough good bacteria left to digest our food. Topping our system up with a daily probiotic in this instance makes a lot of sense. I also recommend probiotics to anyone suffering from irritable bowel syndrome or recurrent thrush.

PROCESSED FOOD, SNACKS AND PORTION SIZES

Having started this chapter naming these three as the main problems with our modern Western diets, and having explained what I mean by a healthy, balanced diet, I need to discuss why these three worry me so much.

- **Processed and pre-packaged foods** – The next time you go shopping and reach for your favourite prepared meal, look at the food label. Even if you don't want to bother with all the numbers, just look at the colours, and remember what I said about the biggest ingredients being at the top of the ingredients list. I know we all lead busy lives and sometimes being able to pop a ready meal in the microwave is very appealing. As an occasional meal, of course, this is perfectly fine. But if your life is so busy that you need to do this several times a week, then I suggest you have a look at some of the healthier options available in supermarkets. These may still be quick to prepare but should be lower in sugar and fat. For example, sachets of lentils or bulgar wheat with roasted vegetables are available in supermarkets, and take just a minute or two to cook in a microwave.

- **Snacks** – It's all too easy to reach for high-calorie (and often high-fat and high-sugar) snacks – and these are often more readily available than others – so you're going to have to plan ahead here. Swapping crisps for nuts or biscuits for dried fruit will undoubtedly be more nutritious. They may still be quite high in calories, though, so try to get into the habit of measuring a portion – and don't go back for more!

- **Portion sizes** – The one good thing I would say about ready meals is that their portion sizes tend to be appropriate. This is important: it's easy to eat a 'meal for two' all on your own. We have simply got used to eating bigger portions and we need to recalibrate our brains. It takes around 20 minutes for chemicals in your stomach to tell your brain that you are full, so my advice is to put all the food you think you are going to eat on the plate and sit down to eat. When you have finished, allow your brain some time to catch up. If you still want seconds 20 minutes later then you can, but how often have you reached for seconds just after finishing a meal, only to feel bloated minutes later and regretting your overindulgence?

DR DAWN'S TOP TIP

If you have chosen to eat a ready meal, try to add a portion (or two or three!) of steamed fresh vegetables to it – and perhaps some fresh fruit as a dessert to make up your five-a-day.

DR DAWN'S TOP TIP

Don't go shopping when you are hungry or feeling a little weak on willpower. If you don't buy unhealthy snacks, they won't be in the kitchen cupboard to tempt you!

DR DAWN'S TOP TIP

Invest in smaller plates and glasses. Your meal will look bigger on a smaller plate and you will feel as though you have had a good meal, but your calorie intake will be dramatically less.

DR DAWN'S TOP TIP

Here's a quirky one to end the chapter with. Don't eat standing up. It's a tip I give many of my patients, and they often ask how standing up affects our metabolism. It doesn't! But the food you eat when standing tends to be either snacks or nibbles with drinks, both of which are unnecessary calories. It is thought that people who graze underestimate their daily calorific intake by between 500 and 1,000 calories! Take time to eat your meals sitting down, and chew your food thoroughly. It takes time for your brain to receive messages from your gut, so if you sit down and take the time to eat your meal you will be less likely to reach for a second helping.

Chapter 6

LET'S GET PHYSICAL

Exercise makes you live longer. OK, maybe I should qualify that statement slightly: people who take regular exercise tend to live longer than those who don't. The evidence is overwhelming, and the health benefits apply to physical exercise or sport of almost every kind. And the really good news is that you don't need to become a fitness fanatic to feel the effects. Just introducing a moderate amount of physical exertion into your daily routine can make a huge difference.

Regular physical exercise has been shown to reduce the risk of cardiovascular disease, stroke, hypertension, type 2 diabetes, osteoporosis, arthritis, obesity, colon cancer, breast cancer, asthma, Alzheimer's disease, erectile dysfunction, chronic pain and even constipation. According to the NHS, this adds up to an overall 30% reduction in the risk of an early death. But if that's not enough of an incentive, consider these additional health benefits:

- Reduced risk of falls, fractures and other injuries from falls. When it comes to your bones, exercise can stimulate bone growth and/or prevent bone loss, and it also improves muscle strength.
- Increased energy levels. Improved blood flow – and the resulting boost in oxygen and nutrient delivery – makes you feel less tired and more energetic.
- Improved management of depression and anxiety disorders. Regular exercise has been shown to help people with mild to

moderate depression, and can be more effective than taking anti-depressant pills.

- Enhanced mental ability. Aerobic exercise appears to increase the size of the hippocampus (the area of your brain responsible for memory and learning). People who keep fit have better cognitive performance, increased creativity and improved problem-solving skills.
- Better sleep. If you go to bed when you're tired after physical exercise, you are less likely to wake early or suffer from insomnia. Physical activity raises the body's core temperature: when it drops back to normal at the end of the day, it signals to your body that it's time to sleep.
- General feeling of well-being and positive outlook. A good workout leads to the release of feel-good chemicals called endorphins. Exercise can boost your self-esteem and reduce stress.
- Stronger immune system. This results in better protection against colds, flu and other common respiratory diseases.
- Better skin. Increased blood flow delivers oxygen and nutrients that are known to improve skin health.
- Reduced risk of disability. Running and aerobic exercise have been shown to postpone the onset of disability in older adults.
- Greater productivity. A study at Leeds Metropolitan University[1] found that office workers who exercise were more productive, more tolerant towards their colleagues, and had better time management skills.
- Finally, exercise can counteract the risk of becoming overweight or obese because it directly offsets the calories consumed in our food. Regular exercise helps you burn fat more efficiently and can lower cholesterol levels.

Best of all, there are virtually no negatives or adverse side-effects associated with exercise. Provided you increase your level of physical fitness gradually, it really is a win–win situation. Dr Mark Tarnopolsky from the University of Ontario has summed it up pretty well: 'If there were a drug that could do for human health everything that exercise can, it would likely be the most valuable pharmaceutical ever developed.'[2]

Statistically, people who are fit do have extended lifespans. A survey of 2,675 Finnish athletes[3] who had competed in the Olympic Games between 1920 and 1965 showed that they lived an average of five and a half years longer than the general population. A similar study of cyclists[4] who had taken part in the Tour de France found an increased life expectancy of eight years.

So if you aren't as fit as you should be, it's time to discover the benefits of this miracle cure – one that is readily available and which can be completely free.

DON'T JUST SIT THERE

Given the overwhelming evidence about the benefits of regular exercise, you'd expect everyone to be busy working out whenever possible. Unfortunately, for most people the reality is somewhat different. We have a very sedentary culture, with many people working at a desk all day and then slouching in front of the TV every evening. All this sitting isn't just unhealthy; it's actually potentially lethal, as a recent American study discovered.

The research, led by Dr Alpa Patel of the American Cancer Society, followed the progress of around 123,000 adults over a 14-year period.[5] All were in good health at the start. She found that men who spent six or more hours each day sitting down had a death rate that was about 20% higher than men who sat for three hours or less. The death rate for women was about 40% higher.

It's even possible to see the effect of sitting too much on the body's cells. Chapter 2 mentioned telomeres, the tiny caps that protect the ends of your DNA. In one group of women who spend most of the day sitting, these telomeres had shortened to the extent that their biological age was almost a decade older than it should have been. Sitting is about as far from exercising as you can get: it burns just one calorie every minute. No wonder the British government's Department of Health describes sitting as the 'silent killer'.

DR DAWN'S TOP TIP

Changing to standing instead of sitting can make a big difference. If you were able to stand at your desk all day, you would actually burn off hundreds more calories than if you remained seated. Some companies make their employees stand up when they have meetings. See if there are opportunities in your daily routine where you could spend at least some of the time standing up.

For the same reason, would you rather work as a train guard or a driver? The guard spends all day standing by the train doors, walking up and down the carriages, and stepping on and off the train at stations. The driver, meanwhile, sits in comfort all day at the front of the train – and is probably much better paid. But (according to research by a leading train operator) train drivers suffer from twice as many fatal heart attacks as guards.

If too much sitting down is bad for you, so is too much sleep. A recent Australian study[6] showed that sleeping nine or more hours every day is potentially fatal. For people who slept this many hours, and who were also sitting for at least six hours a day, the combined effect on mortality figures was the same as smoking.

When it comes to taking exercise, our national record is pretty poor. A study by Bristol University[7] found that one in ten Britons had not even walked continuously for five minutes in the preceding month. Just think what that means. You probably walk to the bus stop or train station on your way to work, or maybe you walk to buy milk at the corner shop. But a tenth of the population (around 4 million adults) doesn't even manage to do that. I'm not sure whether this makes me angry or just sad.

The NHS recommends that adults should do at least 150 minutes per week of moderate activity, or at least 75 minutes per week of vigorous activity. The Bristol study found that only 20% of people achieve this target. It also found that there was a strong link between the amount of exercise taken and different social groups: for example, only 12% of people educated to degree level were found to be physically inactive; those with no qualifications were three times more likely to take little or no exercise.

So, it looks as though Brits are woefully lazy. In the European Union, only Malta and Serbia have a worse record than the UK. Meanwhile, people in the Netherlands put everyone to shame, with around 80% of the adult population taking the recommended level of exercise. Much of this is achieved through 'incidental activity' (that is, they are becoming fit in the course of doing other things, as opposed to exercising for its own sake). In the Netherlands there are more bicycles than there are people, and 71% of adults use their bikes at least once a week.[8]

Modern technology may have made our lives better in many ways, but it has also had a detrimental effect on our level of activity. Our nomadic ancestors had to compete for scarce resources, and to fight or flee from enemies and predators; now any such confrontations only take place on a computer games console. Technology has automated the workplace so that far fewer people are doing manual jobs. Buying food, clothes or household items once required you to leave your home; now you can order almost anything over the internet from the comfort of your sofa. You don't even need to walk across the room to change TV channels any more; for many people, finding the remote control is the most exercise they get.

If you want to live a long and healthy life you need to get fit –

but you need to do it in a way that is practical and achievable, and that fits in with your lifestyle. Too much exercise can be bad; we've all heard stories of middle-aged people who have suddenly decided to go to the gym after years of inactivity, only to drop dead from a heart attack the next day. So start gently, and then build up to the level of exercise that's right for you.

DR DAWN'S TOP TIP

Don't set exercise goals that are too vague. For example, it's fairly meaningless to say 'I'm going to start going to the gym' or 'From now on I'm going to walk more'. You need to be specific: 'I'll go to the gym for 30 minutes, twice a week' or 'I'll walk to work every Thursday'. Then you can easily tell if you're achieving your objective.

It's equally important not to set goals that you will find impossible to achieve. Every New Year people make all sorts of resolutions about swimming two miles every day or running to work every morning. However well-intentioned, most of these plans don't last because they're too ambitious. Start with modest targets, show that you can achieve them, and then you can build up to greater things at a later date.

DON'T LEAVE IT TOO LATE

The younger you start to get fit, the better. I've already mentioned the risk to your health caused by falling over, but for elderly people this is a major problem. The National Institute for Health and Care Excellence (NICE) says that a third of people over 65 fall every year, and a quarter of a million people end up in hospital as a result; of these, 9,000 will die. Falls are the cause of over half of hospital admissions for accidental injury, and they cost the NHS £3.3 billion per year. Hip fracture is the most common serious injury. This accounts for 1.5 million hospital bed days a year; one-third of people who are admitted for a hip fracture will die within a year. (Jimmy

Thirsk, aged 102, who I wrote about at the start of this book, told me that several of his elderly friends have died as a direct result of falls.)

Older bodies can't recover from accidents as easily as young ones do, and once someone has had a bad fall, the psychological consequences can be as severe as the physical ones. People often lose confidence, become fearful, or feel as if they've lost their independence. They may become too afraid to leave their home, making them more socially isolated than they were before. The best way to counteract this is by exercising to build up muscle and bone strength. You can also learn techniques to improve your balance. But if you wait until you're 70 to start exercising, you're going to have to work that much harder to get results.

The UK's Medical Research Council (MRC) found that it was possible to predict who was most likely to die as a result of a fall – years before they reached old age. They showed that two simple tests taken by a group of 5,000 people aged 53 had a powerful correlation with subsequent death rates:[9]

Balance test: Stand on one leg with your eyes closed for 10 seconds. According to the MRC, if you can only manage 2 seconds (or less) you're three times more likely to die in the next 13 years than if you can manage the full 10. (Those who couldn't balance at all were seven times more likely to die!)

Strength test: Stand up from a chair and then sit down again. If you can manage this 35 times or more in a minute, great. But if you can only do this 22 or fewer times a minute, your death rate is statistically doubled.

If you fail either of these tests, you should view it as a warning shot that you need to get fit – and you should make it a priority. In particular, you need to build up your muscle and bone strength.

Resistance exercises such as training with weights are particularly good for this, but most types of sport or fitness activity will be beneficial to some extent.

Elderly people should also make changes to their environment to reduce the risk of a fatal fall. Stairs should be fitted with hand rails, and outside steps can be replaced by ramps. Tripping hazards such as loose rugs and electrical cords should be removed, and there should be bright lighting in corridors and passageways. Skid-resistant mats should be placed in baths and showers. Some people wear hip pads; in the event of a fall, these reduce the risk of a fracture by around 50%.

You should also be aware of other factors that increase your risk of falling. Your eyesight is important, so see the optician regularly and replace your glasses when necessary. Avoid taking any drugs that may cause sudden dizziness. If you have already had a fall, statistically your risk of falling again is greater.

I find it interesting that over the years there have been huge public awareness campaigns to increase road safety, but you never hear about government health initiatives to prevent something as simple and routine as falling over, yet in the UK falls result in around three times as many deaths as road traffic accidents.

FIND YOUR MOTIVATION

It's always easy to find reasons not to do something: 'I'm really tired', 'I've had a long week', 'I just don't feel like it today', 'The weather's really bad,' 'I don't have the willpower', 'There's a good programme on TV'. If this sounds familiar, you're not alone.

Inertia is the enemy of initiative: for every person who has a great business idea, there are 200 others who have a similar idea but who do nothing about it. At a personal level, inertia is what causes people to live in untidy homes, lose contact with friends, fail to meet deadlines, get into debt, underachieve at work, eat junk food, and so on. In most cases inertia is just a kinder word for sloth, which is (according to the Bible) one of the seven deadly sins.

When it comes to exercise, you need to find a way to get motivated. There's a whole industry based on this! Motivational speakers will charge businesses hundreds or thousands of pounds to give advice on how to get people to do things. The best way to overcome inertia is to focus on what you are trying to achieve. With exercise and physical fitness you might draw up a list that goes something like this:

1. I want to feel great and have more energy all the time.

2. I want to lose weight and look fitter.

3. I want to live well to 101!

The exercise routine is your way of getting to these goals. You need to bear your goals in mind every time you put on your sports kit. Stay positive and believe in yourself. Keep telling yourself 'I can do it' – and the chances are that you can.

DR DAWN'S TOP TIP

It can be very helpful to tell friends or family members about your plans – if you do, you're more likely to stick to them. As you progress, your friends and family will also give you support and encouragement; social approval is a powerful incentive to getting results.

If you think you might need extra motivation, and if you're reasonably well off, you could hire a personal trainer. They should have a good knowledge of different sports and activities and what they can achieve for you as an individual. They will provide the motivation you need by setting goals, monitoring your progress and providing feedback. They may also offer advice on other aspects of wellness, such as your general health and nutrition. Either way, if your personal trainer turns up at your door at 7 a.m., you're unlikely to make an excuse and send them away – particularly if you're paying them for their time.

Only a few lifestyle choices can have as great and positive an impact on your health and happiness as physical activity. Irrespective of your age, shape or size, everyone can benefit. However, once you start, you have to keep going. The benefits diminish within just a few weeks if you stop exercising, and it may then be difficult to get back to the level of fitness you had previously achieved. That's one reason why people who have to go into hospital for lengthy periods often take months to get back to a normal life afterwards.

Ultimately you need to make exercise not just part of your daily routine but part of your identity. You will become a different person – one who is fit and healthy. You're likely to feel happier, calmer and have an improved self-image if you're physically active. This is the new you – so what are you waiting for?

EXERCISE YOUR OPTIONS

As you'd expect, different activities require different levels of effort. A woman weighing about 70 kg will burn the following calories in one hour:

Badminton	400
Basketball	475
Bowling	125
Cricket	275
Croquet	100
Cycling (moderate)	400

Football	550
Golf	225
Hockey	475
Horse riding	200
Polo	475
Rugby	600
Running (moderate)	500
Squash	750
Swimming (fast)	600
Table tennis	200
Tennis	400
Volleyball	475[10]

These figures will vary depending on your age, weight and current level of fitness. If you look online, you'll find lots of websites that let you calculate the calorie count for hundreds of different sports and activities. (Having sex may be a pleasurable alternative to anything listed above – this works out at around 200 calories per hour!)

DR DAWN'S TOP TIP

If you start a programme of regular sport or exercise in the hope of losing lots of weight, it may take some time before you see any results. This is partly because muscle tissue is denser and heavier than fat so, as you burn calories through exercise, your muscle should be increasing as your fat decreases. At first you may not see much difference when you stand on the scales, but that doesn't mean the exercise isn't already doing you some good. That's why swapping the scales for a tape measure may give you more encouragement that you are getting results.

Your choice of sport or activity will depend on many factors. You probably need to be tall to be good at basketball, and you'll need high levels of endurance to enjoy a triathlon. Similarly, you may prefer to do your own thing by going to the gym, or you may prefer the sociable element of a team game. Cost and time are important considerations. There may be a fantastic new gym in your nearest country club, but you'll be asked to pay a substantial membership fee and sign a contract that's very hard to get out of. And there's no point joining a football team if your existing commitments make it impossible to play or practise on a regular basis.

Depending on what you want to achieve, you should consider whether you want to do aerobic or anaerobic exercise. Aerobic ('with oxygen') exercise includes any type of activity that maintains an increased heart rate, and is usually performed at a moderately high level of intensity over a long period of time. It's the type where you get out of breath in just a few moments. So, for example, running a long distance at a moderate pace is aerobic exercise, whereas weight lifting is anaerobic. Aerobic exercise is good for burning lots of calories to reduce fat; it also strengthens the muscles, including the all-important heart muscles. Anaerobic exercise can help you build a lean, toned body and increase your physical endurance. Most activities can be either aerobic or anaerobic, depending on how hard you're exerting yourself.

You may complain that you don't have enough time to incorporate any kind of exercise regime into your busy life. I would say that you can always find time to do something that matters to you – and being fit really matters in the long run. It may be that you have to sacrifice something else in order to get fit, such as time spent watching TV or chatting online with friends.

DR DAWN'S TOP TIP

You could try keeping an hour-by-hour diary of a typical week to see where your time goes. You might find that you're wasting several hours on things that aren't important.

Many people choose to exercise first thing in the morning because it's less likely that other things will get in the way. (I have noticed that whenever a newspaper has a 'day in the life' feature about a successful business person, they always get up at around 5 a.m. and head to the gym!) This also has the advantage of making you feel good first thing in the morning, setting you up for the day ahead. Exercising at lunchtime may be a more practical alternative, particularly if there's a gym near your place of work.

If you're simply too busy during the working week to do any exercise, all is not lost. A recent study carried out by Loughborough University[11] looked at people who describe themselves as 'weekend warriors'. These are people who are fairly inactive from Monday to Friday, but who then make up for it by playing tennis or pounding the pavements at weekends. The study followed the progress of 63,000 people over a decade. It found that even having an irregular pattern of exercise, people in this group were 30% less likely to die during the 10-year period than people who did no exercise at all. Loughborough's Dr Gary O'Donovan said: 'One of the most surprising findings was that doing one or two bouts of activity a week, even if you don't meet the recommended volumes, is beneficial.' In other words, even if your lifestyle restricts your ability to exercise at certain times of the week, it doesn't matter. As long as you can catch up at other times (aiming for that NHS target, if possible), you'll still get the benefits.

Whatever time you choose and however much exercise you manage to do, there are plenty of different ways you can get fit, so it's a matter of finding a sport or activity that works for you. You could amaze your friends by doing something outlandish or different. Remember, you're aiming for the NHS recommended activity level of at least 150 minutes of moderate aerobic activity (such as cycling or fast walking) every week, and strength exercises on two or more days a week.

Here are a few quirky ideas from around the world:

Chess boxing – Popular in parts of Germany, this is (as you would expect) a combination of chess and boxing, requiring both brains and brawn.

Dog dancing – Also known as canine freestyle, this is a competitive sport in which owners dance with their favourite pets. Popular in Japan.

Ostrich racing – You sit on your favourite ostrich and race around a track at speeds of up to 43 miles an hour. Originating in Africa, it now also has a following in the USA.

Quidditch – Taken from the pages of Harry Potter into real life, the game has the same rules and scoring system as in the book – but without the flying.

Buzkashi – A variant of polo, but one in which the normal wooden mallet is replaced by the carcass of a cow or goat. The team that drags the carcass across the opposing team's goal line wins. Popular in Central Asia.

Alternatively, you could start with something that's readily available and costs you nothing – walking.

PUT YOUR BEST FOOT FORWARD

The simple act of walking will make you healthier and it could add years to your life. Recent studies have shown remarkable results. Just half an hour a day of moderately paced walking can cut your risk of having a fatal heart attack by half. Walking is also just as good as running for reducing high blood pressure and cholesterol.

People who walk a lot have been found to have lower BMIs and smaller waists than many people who take part in more vigorous exercises. Also, the more time you spend walking, the less time you spend sitting – which, as we have already seen, is bad for you.

Adding a stroll to your daily routine is more important than ever

– or you could simply make an effort to walk wherever possible. A friend of mine who works in London decided to do just that. He is a publicist, so he has to travel round the city to meetings most days – but a year ago he decided he would walk to meetings. Using an app on his phone, he now tries to walk at least 10,000 steps each day (about 5 miles, or 8 kilometres). He says the benefits have been amazing – he's lost weight and feels great. As an incidental bonus, he's saved a fortune on train tickets and taxi fares, and avoided the frustration of being stuck in traffic jams.

Walking burns 200–250 calories per hour. It helps to strengthen the muscles in your legs and buttocks. As you walk, each stride also stresses your bones in a positive way so that more bone tissue is created. You'll also find a lot of the other benefits of doing exercise listed at the start of this chapter. Professor Greg Whyte from Liverpool John Moores University summed it up like this: 'Substituting one hour of sitting with one hour of walking results in a 13% drop in all-cause mortality. You live longer [and] the mental benefits of walking are phenomenal.'[12]

DR DAWN'S TOP TIP

Build up to your target distance gradually; if you over-exert yourself too soon, you may find it too stressful and give up. Once you've reached a distance you're comfortable with, you can try adding short bursts of fast walking into your routine, or you could incorporate the occasional hill into your route. Walking uphill typically burns off about 60% more calories than walking on a flat surface.

The NHS recommends walking as the easiest way of trying to reach the government's recommended target of 150 minutes of moderate exercise a week. You can increase the amount you walk by doing so at every opportunity. In a survey carried out in August 2017, Public Health England found that four out of ten middle-aged adults in the UK don't walk briskly for 10 minutes in any one month![13] Walking briskly for 10 minutes just once a day reduces the risk of heart disease and type 2 diabetes by 40%. Public Health England has developed an app called Active 10. You carry your phone with you in a pocket or a handbag, and the app tells you at the end of each day how many minutes you have walked and how many of those were brisk walking. You can set your target for 10, 20 or 30 minutes per day. Public Health England thinks this app will really help all those people who say they haven't got time to exercise, as 10 minutes per day is achievable for everyone! I've been using the app,[14] and it has made me walk more quickly around London – I have found that I can get from one office I work in regularly to Paddington in half an hour, which is how long it used to take me on the Tube!

Also, as I mentioned in Chapter 4 on diabetes, I decided to increase the amount of walking I did every day by walking to the waiting room to call my patients in rather than using an intercom system. There are lots of small changes you could make to your daily routine to increase your step count and enhance the health benefits:

- Walk to work. If the journey is too far, consider getting off the train or bus a stop earlier and walking the rest of the way.
- Always try to use the stairs instead of the lift. Climbing stairs burns more calories per minute than swimming, cycling or tennis!
- Walk up escalators. It's quicker, and you can get that sense of superiority as you stride past (often younger) people who are taking the lazy option by standing.
- Get a dog. Most dogs need regular walks, and your dog looking soulfully at you will encourage you to get up and walk them. You will also meet other dog walkers and will make new friends.
- If you do the same journey regularly (e.g. walking to work), start to vary your route to stop yourself getting bored.
- If you have children, walk them to school if possible. You will then also be instilling good habits in them.
- Plan interesting walks to enjoy on days off. There are dozens of books that give detailed itineraries, both in rural and urban areas.

There are also various websites from which you can download suggested walks with detailed maps.

- If you have a car, resolve not to use it for any journey where you could just as easily walk (e.g. under a mile). If you're in a city, you could find that by the time you've crawled through the traffic and found a parking space, it's probably quicker to walk anyway.
- If you find that walking can get a bit boring, you could explore ways to make things more interesting. You can listen to music or, as I sometimes do, set yourself a mental exercise – for example, to find a solution to a work problem.

Sir Edward Elgar was one of Britain's greatest classical composers. He used to set off on long walks along the Malvern Hills in Worcestershire, forming new compositions in his head. Then he would return home each evening to write them down. 'This music is what I hear all day,' he said. 'The trees are singing my music – or have I sung theirs?' (Note: Elgar lived to the age of 76, which was well above the average for someone born in 1857.)

You can make walking more sociable by finding a partner, such as a colleague who has a similar route to work. Just as with hiring a personal trainer, you're less likely to find an excuse not to walk if the arrangement involves someone else. Or you can participate in organised group walks, such as those arranged by the Ramblers, the UK's walking association. If you're really ambitious, you could sign up for a long-distance charity walk – trekking across the Himalayas would really increase your fitness level, and you'd be raising money for a good cause in the process.

These days you can also use technology to enhance your walking experience. There's a huge range of fitness watches that will track steps, distance, calories burned and vertical ascents or descents for any journey, and there are a number of apps – many of them free – that you can use on your phone. Here are four, as recommended by the British Heart Foundation:

MapMyWalk: this app tracks your route, time, distance, speed pace and calories burned.

OutDoors Great Britain: this gives you access to a variety of free maps that you can store on your phone, so that you can see where you're going even when you don't have internet access. You can also pay to upload the full range of Ordnance Survey maps.

ViewRanger: another app that gives you access to free and/or paid for maps. This one lets you plan routes on your computer and then access them on your phone. You can also import and export walking routes to share them with other people.

World Walking: like many other apps, this records the number of steps you take each day. But you can also choose a legendary route, such as Route 66 in the USA or Peru's Machu Picchu Inca Trail, and then try to take enough steps to complete it (cool!).

Walking offers another important benefit. Unless you're achieving all your step count on a treadmill, you're going to be spending more time outdoors, which means you're exposed to sunlight, which stimulates your body to produce vitamin D (see Chapter 5). And of course being in the great outdoors has additional benefits. Fresh air, sunshine and greenery can all play their part in helping you to de-stress and improve your mood. You'll feel more alive, energetic and optimistic.

YOU SHOULD BE DANCING

Here's another interesting – and enjoyable – way to get physically fit. Scientists at the University of Magdeburg in Germany were able to show that dancing can be more effective than going to the gym.[15] They took a group of 57 healthy people, aged 65–80, and split them into two groups. One group was given dance training for 90 minutes, twice a week. The other group spent the same amount of time doing aerobic exercises in the gym.

After six months, the dancers were found to be measurably fitter and they had visibly more grey matter in their brains than the gym-goers. Or, as the research concluded, 'Multimodal stimulation and the continuous learning associated with dancing is more effective than monotonic physical exercise.' Of course!

A study carried out at the University of Brighton[16] found similarly positive results when testing the effects of dancing on a group of much younger people (aged from 24 to 38). The dancers wore vests that could measure their heart rate and their energy expenditure. They then attended a variety of half-hour dance classes. The dancers in contemporary, street and swing dance classes burned more calories than they would have done running or cycling for the same period. Swing dancing was the most effective, burning 586 calories per hour. Even ballet dancing scored well as it was shown to include periods of 'high and severe intensity exercise'.

So dance is a fun and sociable way to keep fit, and it's readily accessible to most people. Next time you see a group of elderly people at a 'tea dance', you'll realise that, although it may look very genteel, they are actually doing their bodies a lot of good in the process.

MARATHON MAN

Exercise is good for you, however old you are. If you can keep exercising into old age, you'll continue to enjoy the benefits and you could be as fit as someone much younger.

Fauja Singh (known as the 'Turbaned Tornado') from Ilford in East London has become the oldest marathon runner in the world. He started long-distance running when he was 81, and took part in his first marathon at the age of 89. He completed the 26.2-mile course in 6 hours and 54 minutes, knocking almost an hour off the record for someone of his age.

He went on to become the first centenarian to run in a marathon, completing the Toronto Waterfront Marathon in 8 hours and 11 minutes. Although he announced his retirement from marathons at the age of 101, he still continues to run shorter distances. 'The day I stop running, my body will stop altogether and that will be the end of me,' he said. Fauja Singh was awarded the British Empire Medal in the 2015 New Year's Honours list. He recently celebrated his 106th birthday.

DR DAWN'S TOP TIP

Although most types of exercise are beneficial for most people, you should talk to your doctor before starting a new fitness programme if you suffer from any of the following:

- asthma or lung disease
- type 1 or type 2 diabetes
- heart disease, or the possibility that you may have a heart problem
- arthritis
- kidney disease
- dizzy spells or unsteadiness on your feet
- you are undergoing treatment for any other serious or chronic condition.

CHAPTER 7

A HEALTHY HEART

Initially, this chapter was going to be about heart disease. Cancer may feature in more headlines, but heart disease remains one of the biggest killers in the UK, taking over 80,000 lives prematurely each year. One in six men and one in ten women in the UK will die from heart disease: there are 2.3 million people living with heart disease in the UK today, and two million affected by angina, which impacts their quality of life.

But the more I thought about this chapter, the more I realised that what we need to address is how to keep our arteries healthy, because it's not just heart disease that can take us when we're young. Each year, 152,000 Brits have a stroke – that's one every 3 minutes, 27 seconds – and, of those, one in eight die within a month, and one in four die within a year. Half of all stroke survivors are left with a permanent disability. By the age of 75, one in six men and one in five women will have had a stroke. Those are scary statistics, but the good news is that there's a lot we can do to ensure the same does not happen to us.

I am also going to talk about dementia in this chapter, because there are over 850,000 people living with dementia in the UK today and numbers are rising – by so much that experts are predicting we could have more than one million people with dementia in the UK by 2025. Vascular dementia occurs when veins and arteries that supply blood to the brain become blocked or narrowed.

CORONARY HEART DISEASE

The heart is a four-chambered muscular organ that requires a good blood supply to work efficiently. It gets its blood supply from the coronary arteries, which are the first to branch off the aorta as it leaves the left ventricle. If those blood vessels get furred up, the blood supply to the heart muscle (or myocardium) is compromised. This is called coronary heart disease (CHD), or ischaemic heart disease, and may cause symptoms of angina or a heart attack.

Our heart is the pump that sends fuel to the rest of the body. It beats over 100,000 times every day.

WHAT IS A HEART ATTACK?

In a heart attack, the blood supply to part of the heart is cut off, causing the muscle supplied by that vessel to die. A heart attack is also sometimes called a myocardial infarction (MI) – myocardial, meaning heart muscle, and infarction, meaning dead tissue.

A person experiencing a heart attack (or MI) usually has a central crushing chest pain, which may radiate into the left arm, neck or jaw. Sometimes they feel pain in both arms – or there may be no pain, but the attack is picked up on an ECG tracing. (An ECG is an electrocardiogram: it shows the electrical activity of the heart. It is used to diagnose angina, heart attacks and heart rhythm problems.) The pain may be associated with shortness of breath, feeling sick or light-headed. You may feel clammy and those around you may think you look pale or grey. This is a medical emergency and you, or someone near you, should call 999 immediately.

The most common cause of a heart attack is a clot blocking an artery. The size and severity of the heart attack depends on the size of the blood vessel that is blocked. If a small artery is blocked, then a small area of muscle will be affected and you are less likely to have long-term problems. If one of the main coronary arteries is blocked, then a large part of the muscle is affected and, unless the blood vessel can be opened again quickly, you are likely to be left short of breath on minimal exertion, because the heart can't pump hard enough with the healthy muscle that is left. This can be seriously disabling – I have met far too many people who are housebound due to heart problems. If we are going to live well until 101 years, we need to look after our arteries.

There are some things that increase our risk of a heart attack that we can do nothing about. These include:

- **age** – most heart attacks occur in the over-50s.
- **gender** – men are more at risk than premenopausal women, as oestrogen protects the heart. After the menopause, the risk for women starts to increase.
- **ethnicity** – Asian and Afro-Caribbean people are more at risk than Caucasians.
- **family history** – if your father or brother had coronary heart disease or a thrombotic stroke (a stroke caused by a blood clot rather than a stroke caused by a bleed. Clinically, the strokes look the same, but diagnosis is made on a scan) before the age of 55, or your mother or sister before the age of 60, this is deemed to be a positive family history and increases your risk.
- **type 1 diabetes** – this is a condition in which your body produces antibodies to itself, and the pancreas cannot produce enough insulin to maintain healthy blood sugar levels. It is associated with a significant increased risk of developing coronary artery disease.

There are significant other risk factors that we can – and should – do something about, and they are down to our lifestyles. They include:

- **Smoking** – the more you smoke, the greater the risk. It is thought that 20% of deaths from coronary artery disease in men, and 17% in women, are due to smoking; but the good news is that you can reduce your risk by 25% if you stop smoking. Once you have given up for 15 years, your risk returns to that of a non-smoker!

- **Obesity** – a high-fat diet increases your risk, and it is thought that as many as a third of all CHD deaths are due to poor diet. The risk is highest when excess weight is carried around the middle. If you take two identical women, same height and same weight – one woman carries weight around her middle (apple-shaped) and the other carries her weight around her hips and thighs (pear-shaped) – the apple-shaped woman would have a greater risk of developing heart disease than the pear-shaped woman.

DR DAWN'S TOP TIP

Measure your waist today. To measure your waist, you need to feel for your hip bone and for the bottom of your ribs, and breathe out naturally (don't force your abdomen out, just gently exhale) then measure your circumference midway between these two points. It is always a good idea to check the measurement more than once to check that you have done this accurately. Women should have a waistline no greater than 80 cm (31.5 inches) and men no greater than 94 cm (37 inches). Waistlines greater than this are associated with significantly increased risk of high blood pressure, heart disease and diabetes. If you are of Asian descent, things get even tougher – Asian men are at increased risk, so the numbers are smaller – your waistlines should be no more than 90 cm (35.5 inches).

- **Lack of exercise** – you should aim to exercise for at least 30 minutes at least five times a week, and that's on top of the recommended 10,000 steps a day.
- **Hypertension** – blood pressure should be 140/90 or lower to prevent strain on the heart.
- **Cholesterol** – cholesterol is implicated in nearly half of all cardiac deaths. If everyone in the country had a total cholesterol

of less than 6.5 mmol/l, then we could reduce all deaths from coronary artery disease by 10%.

- **Type 2 diabetes** – not only does type 2 diabetes increase your risks, but it magnifies the effect of other risk factors.
- **Alcohol** – consistently drinking more than the recommended 14 units per week increases your risk of coronary heart disease, and binge drinking is thought to be the most risky.

DR DAWN'S TOP TIP

Invest in a pedometer – I know I have said this before, but when you start counting your steps, you may discover that you are not as active as you thought and you need to look at ways of increasing your activity (which are achievable and sustainable) to keep your heart healthy.

DR DAWN'S TOP TIP

Factor in at least two dry days every week to reduce your total alcohol intake. This year we have a new house rule: we have promised ourselves that we won't drink alcohol at home during the week. It is all too easy to pour a glass or two every night with supper, but this is a simple and easily achievable rule that will go a long way to looking after our hearts.

STROKE

A stroke occurs when the blood supply to the brain is cut off. In eight out of ten cases this is due to a blood clot, which forms in an area of narrowed artery, usually due to atherosclerosis. Our arteries harden as we age, but there are several lifestyle factors (which I will discuss in this chapter) that can speed up that process; conversely, if we address those factors and alter our lifestyle, we can reduce our risk. Given that there are over 150,000 strokes every year in the UK, and that stroke is the commonest cause of adult disability worldwide, this is something we should take seriously. My late grandmother suffered a stroke, and it was sad to see such a vibrant woman become incapacitated and dependent in her later years.

TRANSIENT ISCHAEMIC ATTACK

A transient ischaemic attack (TIA) is often referred to as a mini stroke. They have the same symptoms as a stroke but the patient recovers more quickly – sometimes within minutes, but always within 24 hours.

One in three people who suffer a TIA will have a stroke at some point in the following year, so it is important that we recognise what is happening and do all we can to reduce that risk. One in six people who have had a TIA will go on to have a heart attack. Reducing the risk of these events is about doing the things that reduce your risk of a stroke generally, and taking any medication prescribed by your doctor.

HOW CAN YOU TELL IF YOU ARE GOING TO BE ONE OF THE UNLUCKY ONES?

The simple answer is you can't. None of us have a crystal ball, but doctors use a scoring system to try to identify those people who have had a stroke and are most at risk of having another. This is called the ABCD score:

- **Age** – being over 60 = 1 point
- **Blood pressure** – greater than 140 systolic or 90 diastolic = 1 point
- **Clinical features** – one-sided weakness = 2 points, and speech difficulties = 1 point

- **D**uration of symptoms – greater than one hour = 2 points, and 10–59 minutes = 1 point
- **D**iabetes, if present = 1 point.

A score of less than 4 is low risk, but if you score over 6, then you have a significant risk of developing a stroke during the following week.

HYPERTENSION

Hypertension is the medical term for high blood pressure. Blood pressure is the pressure created in the arteries as blood is pumped out of the heart. It is usually measured, while sitting, from the brachial artery – the artery you can feel pulsating in the crease of your elbow. It is completely appropriate for blood pressure to be raised when you are exercising or in pain. It is also normal for blood pressure to go up when you are stressed. In evolutionary terms, this is a good thing. It was a response to an adrenalin rush, which is part of the fight or flight reaction. If a mammoth is looming, it's a good thing that you are wired and alert, and ready to run or stand and fight. The problem today is that our stresses don't come in the form of an occasional mammoth. They are more likely to be daily pressures, such as meeting deadlines, relationship problems, or juggling family and work.

You can feel perfectly well with high blood pressure. Contrary to popular belief, most people do; they don't have headaches or blurred vision. Most people have no idea that they are at risk unless they are checked. I think that everyone over 40 should know their blood pressure. I am rarely concerned about a one-off high reading, unless it is extremely high. Consistently high blood pressure will put a strain on your heart. Your heart is a bit like a car engine. If you occasionally put your foot on the throttle to accelerate past a 'mammoth', your engine (heart) will cope fine. But if you spend your life with your foot on the floor (everyday stress and pressure) eventually your engine (heart) will start to show the strain.

That is why we rarely diagnose hypertension after a one-off reading. If your doctor or nurse notices that your blood pressure is raised, they will repeat this once or twice, and may ask you to return on different days to gather a selection of readings.

DR DAWN'S TOP TIP

If you are over 40 (or younger, but have a family history of heart disease), make an appointment to see your practice nurse or visit a local pharmacy that offers the service and get your blood pressure checked.

Many surgeries also use home blood pressure monitors and will ask you to take several readings at home with an electronic monitor at different times of the day to rule out 'white coat hypertension'. This refers to people who always have high blood pressure readings when they are sitting in front of a doctor, but whose home readings are normal. The term comes from the days when doctors wore white coats. It is a surprisingly common phenomenon, and why many doctors use home monitors or special machines that record your blood pressure for 24 hours or more. If you can prove that your blood pressure is only raised when you are sitting in the consulting room, but that your measurements are fine at home, then it is unlikely that you will need treatment. I generally ask people to take a couple of readings each day, at different times of the day, for a couple of weeks, and then bring in the results. I also ask them to bring their monitor so that we can compare the readings in the surgery. If the home monitor agrees with my sphygmomanometer, then I know I can rely on the home readings.

HOW HIGH IS TOO HIGH?

Blood pressure is recorded as two numbers – the systolic value is the higher pressure that the system reaches, and the diastolic value is the lower pressure. Normal blood pressure is less than 140/90. If your blood pressure is consistently 160/100 or more, then you will almost certainly need medication. If it is between 140/90 and 160/100, your GP may suggest some changes to your lifestyle to try to reduce your blood pressure before starting you on pills. If you are diabetic, or already have kidney or heart problems, your doctor will probably aim for your blood pressure to be lower, at 130/80.

WHAT CAUSES HIGH BLOOD PRESSURE?

In most cases, there is no one specific cause of high blood pressure. This is called essential hypertension and shows how hard the heart is pumping, and how much resistance there is in the arteries, which is caused by narrowing of the arteries.

Sometimes, there is an identifiable cause for high blood pressure, such as kidney disease or hormonal problems, and in this case it is referred to as secondary hypertension.

About half of adults over 65 in the UK have high blood pressure, and it is more common in those with diabetes and people of Afro-Caribbean or Asian descent, or in people who have close relatives with high blood pressure.

Being overweight, smoking, drinking too much alcohol, eating too much salt and being inactive all increase the likelihood of having high blood pressure.

WHAT CAN I DO TO LOWER MY BLOOD PRESSURE?

There are several lifestyle changes that can influence your blood pressure and reduce your risk of a heart attack or stroke:

• **Smoking** – If you are a smoker, you should stop now. Smoking doesn't necessarily cause high blood pressure but it adds to your risk of developing heart disease. Your GP and pharmacist will be able to help you.

- **Weight** – If you are overweight, you should aim to lose weight gradually – one to two pounds a week until you have a healthy BMI. You can calculate your BMI by dividing your weight in kilos by the square of your height in metres. If I am 1.63 m tall and weigh 52 kg, my BMI is: BMI = $52/(1.63 \times 1.63)$ = 19.5. A healthy BMI is between 18.5 and 25. Even a small weight loss can make a big difference – a 1-kg loss can equate to a fall in blood pressure of 2.5/1.5. See the BMI chart on page 80.

- **Diet** – If you have high blood pressure, it is important that you address your diet and aim to have a healthy well-balanced diet (this is covered in detail in Chapter 5), but if you do nothing else, watch your fat intake – remember only a third of your total calories should be fat, and of these you should limit your intake of trans fats and saturated fats to a third of your total fat intake.

- **Salt** – We are used to a high salt diet in the Western world. You should limit your daily intake to 6 grams. When you start to look at the hidden salt in processed foods, you will be shocked by the amounts.

- **Exercise** – You should aim to do half an hour of exercise at least five times a week. It doesn't matter what you do. It doesn't have to be in a fancy gym, but you should choose something you enjoy doing so you will stick with it. It's even better if you exercise with a friend, then you will encourage each other when your willpower is weak. Whether it's a brisk walk, cycling, jogging, swimming or dancing, you need to be exercising at a level that makes you out of breath. If you are gasping for breath, then you should ease back a bit, but if you can chat easily while you are doing your exercise, then you need to up your game!

- **Alcohol** – Drinking to excess can lead to an increase in blood pressure, so make sure you stick to recommended limits for alcohol of 14 units per week.

- **Caffeine** – The effect that caffeine has on blood pressure is small, but if you have high blood pressure, then it is a good idea to restrict your intake to five caffeinated drinks per day.

DR DAWN'S TOP TIP

Swap your coffee at home for a decaffeinated variety to reduce your total caffeine intake.

CHOLESTEROL

Cholesterol is a fat or lipid, which is partly made in cells in our body and partly derived from the food that we eat. Contrary to popular belief, not all cholesterol is bad; we need some cholesterol to stay healthy. When we measure cholesterol, we measure the total cholesterol, but we also look at the levels of different lipoprotein that circulate in the bloodstream. As the name suggests, these compounds are a combination of protein and lipid. This is the way cholesterol is transported in the bloodstream. There are several different lipoproteins, but those relevant to cholesterol are low density lipoproteins (LDLs) and high density lipoproteins (HDLs). The LDLs are often referred to as 'bad' cholesterol and the HDLs as 'good' cholesterol. The LDLs comprise most of the cholesterol. If you are diabetic, or have already been diagnosed with heart disease, your doctor will want to reduce your total cholesterol level, but if you are at risk of developing heart disease, they will be more interested in the ratio of your good cholesterol to the total level.

WHAT IS NORMAL CHOLESTEROL?

Cholesterol is measured in the blood in mmol per litre (mmol/l). Total cholesterol should be less than 5.0 mmol/l, LDL cholesterol should be less than 3 mmol/l and HDL cholesterol more than 1.2 mmol/l.

Generally, the lower your LDL and the higher your HDL, the better. We often look at the ratio of total cholesterol to HDL. Total cholesterol, divided by HDL, should ideally be less than 4.5 but whether or not your doctor decides to treat your cholesterol will depend on other risk factors for heart disease, such as your age, gender, blood pressure and whether or not you smoke.

HOW CAN I TELL IF MY CHOLESTEROL IS HIGH?

Occasionally, a high cholesterol level will cause yellow waxy-looking plaques in the skin around the eyes, called xanthelasma, or fatty lumps on the elbows, called xanthomas. But in most cases, there is no obvious outside sign that your cholesterol is high, and the only way to find out is to have a blood test. Some chemists offer a pinprick test, which gives you an idea of your total cholesterol. If you have a test like this, which suggests your level is high, your GP will want to do a formal blood test. These are usually done on a fasting sample. (That means having nothing to eat or drink for eight hours before the blood test.)

DR DAWN'S TOP TIP

If you are over 40, or have a family history of heart disease or stroke at a young age, don't leave things to chance – make an appointment to have your cholesterol checked so you can do something about it before it is too late.

HOW CAN MY CHOLESTEROL BE HIGH IF I EAT HEALTHILY?

Only about 10–20% of your total cholesterol comes from what you eat. The rest is made by your body, and is genetically predetermined. That is why it is possible to find fat people who eat a high cholesterol diet, but have low cholesterol in their bloodstream, and others who eat healthily but have high cholesterol, because their bodies make more of it.

WHY DOES CHOLESTEROL MATTER?

We need some cholesterol in our body – for example, it is the substance that is found in cell walls – but high levels of cholesterol can cause fatty plaques to form on the walls of the blood vessels. Over time these plaques can build up and harden, forming atherosclerosis, or hardening of the arteries. This can mean that not enough blood is being delivered to certain parts of the body. If the plaques form in the coronary arteries, this causes heart disease. If they form in the blood vessels supplying the brain, they can cause strokes, and if they form in the vessels in the legs, they can cause severe pain when walking, which is called claudication.

Sometimes blood clots form on the plaques, and if they break off, they can then block an artery, which means no blood can get through, and this can lead to a heart attack, stroke or gangrene.

It is thought that high cholesterol is implicated in half of all heart attacks.

DEMENTIA

Human memory is immensely complex and precious. Most weeks I see someone concerned that they are losing their memory. I often describe our memory as a *suitcase*. We are born with an empty suitcase and throughout our lives we put things in that case. When it is relatively empty, it is easy to put in new things, but as it gets full there is less space. Eventually it is full to bursting and every time we try to put something new in, something else must be displaced. When we lose our memory, it is our memories of recent events (the things we have only just placed in the suitcase) that go. If you spend some time talking to anyone with dementia, they may have no idea what they had for lunch an hour ago, or whether they had lunch, or what day it is, but they may be able to remember their wedding day, or wartime experiences, in minute detail.

It is normal to become forgetful with age, and I try to reassure people it is completely normal to forget where you put your car keys. What is not normal is to forget what they are for, or to find that you have put them in the fridge or your sock drawer!

WHICH PART OF THE BRAIN CONTROLS MEMORY?

There is no one part of the brain that is responsible for memory. We have all heard people talk about the fact that once you have learned how to do it, you never forget how to ride a bike. I once heard a doctor give a lecture on this to illustrate how complex memory is. To ride a bike, you need to remember how you physically balance on it and move the pedals, you need to remember the route to take from A to B, and you need to remember the Highway Code – to make sure you are safe on the roads and look out for other road users. These memories all involve different parts of the brain.

When we remember events, we need to retrieve the information from our memory bank, and this is done in one of two ways. First, short-term memory is retrieved sequentially. If someone reads a limerick and then asks you to repeat the third line, you will read through the limerick in your head (or out loud) to retrieve the information. Second, long-term memory is stored and retrieved by association, which is why you may find yourself feeling emotional about a song before you have consciously remembered its significance. This is also why, when you go into the kitchen to get something and can't remember what you were looking for, if you go back to the first room you were in, that often triggers your memory.

WHAT CAUSES MEMORY LOSS?

There are lots of things that cause loss of memory, and often it is that you weren't concentrating when the information went in. If you are reading a newspaper when someone asks you to phone the window cleaner, you may well not remember. That's not because you are losing your mind; it's because you weren't listening at the time and it wasn't a priority. If, on the same day, you were reading the same newspaper and were offered tickets to see your favourite band play live, you would remember, because you would have shifted your focus of attention.

Other factors that influence our memory include:

- **Age** – we are more forgetful as we get older. That is not the same as dementia. It's just that our suitcases are full.
- **Mental health problems** – stress, anxiety and depression affect our ability to concentrate and may affect memory.
- **Drugs** – any drug that has a sedating side-effect can impair your ability to remember. If you think your memory is going downhill since starting a new medication, discuss it with your GP. Don't be tempted to stop taking a prescribed drug without talking to your doctor, but do talk to them, as there may well be an alternative that you find more acceptable.
- **Head injury** – minor head injuries can cause short-term memory problems, but more significant injuries may cause longer-term issues.
- **Stroke** – depending on the part of the brain affected, you may have memory problems after a stroke.
- **Brain tumour** – depending on the part of the brain affected, you may have memory problems after a brain tumour.
- **Alcohol** – drinking excessively in a binge may mean you can't remember what happened the following morning, and alcoholics are also at risk of long-term memory problems.

- **Hypothyroidism** – an underactive thyroid can leave you feeling lethargic and excessively sleepy, which affects your memory.
- **Infections** – particularly in the elderly, a chest or urine infection may cause confusion and memory problems.

DR DAWN'S TOP TIP

It doesn't matter what it is, but do something every day to exercise your brain. Even a few minutes each day will reap rewards. Let's face it, nobody wants to make it to 101 years but then have no idea what is going on around them.

If you know you are getting forgetful, write things down, set alarms for yourself, and try to set up a routine so that you know where you put things.

I am often asked about gingko biloba supplements. It is thought to work by improving blood flow to the brain. Research studies don't all agree, but it may be worth a try. It doesn't seem to work as a preventative cure for dementia, but it may help to boost memory. As with any herbal remedy, I have two simple rules. The first is always tell your doctor if you are taking a herbal remedy, as it may interfere with some conventional medicines. Gingko, for example, has blood-thinning properties. The other rule is to choose a preparation that has a patient information leaflet in the packaging. Herbal remedies are not as tightly regulated as medicines, but some manufacturers volunteer to have their products regulated and these products will have a leaflet inside, so you know what you are getting.

WHAT IS DEMENTIA?

Dementia is the most serious form of memory loss and the one that people worry most about. It is progressive, although variable in the way it progresses.

Dementia is most common in the elderly, but can affect anyone. I have met young, previously mentally agile people whose lives have been wrecked by the condition. Your risk of dementia is increased by:

- cardiovascular risk factors – high blood pressure, high cholesterol, diabetes, obesity, smoking and lack of exercise will increase your risk of developing dementia – and not just vascular (or multi-infarct) dementia, but all types
- Parkinson's disease
- head injury
- family history
- mental health problems – severe depression and schizophrenia can increase your risk
- low IQ and/or learning disabilities.

WHAT ARE THE MAIN TYPES OF DEMENTIA?

The three main types of dementia are:

- **Alzheimer's disease** – this disease is named after the doctor who first described the condition. Alzheimer's is a progressive loss of memory and brain function, and the most common form of dementia. There are more than 520,000 people living with dementia in the UK. Proteins build up in the brain and prevent the normal electrical messages getting through. Ultimately, this leads to the death of nerve cells and loss of brain matter. There is also a shortage of the chemicals that are used to pass messages between nerves in the brain. In the early stages of the disease, individuals may seem forgetful. They may forget a special birthday, or what you were just talking about but, as the disease progresses, they may find it difficult to follow a conversation. They may forget to turn the oven off, or that they have left the front door wide open. This can be frustrating, and emotions can manifest as outbursts of aggression. Eventually, the person becomes unable to care for themselves and needs 24-hour care and supervision. I am often asked how long this process takes. Unfortunately, it is impossible to tell. Some people decline gradually over many years and other people experience a faster deterioration. According to the global deterioration scale for assessment of primary degenerative dementia, it can take from 3.5 to 6 years from diagnosis to when an individual becomes dependent on others for most of their care.[1]

• **Vascular (multi-infarct) dementia** – vascular dementia is caused by mini strokes in the brain, and clinically it differs from Alzheimer's. Rather than a gradual decline in mental function, you are more likely to see a stepwise demise (sudden changes, which may be large or small) with each mini stroke.

• **Lewy body dementia** – Lewy body is named after the abnormal protein deposits that are found in this form of dementia. It may present in the same way as Alzheimer's or vascular dementia, but if the deposits are formed in the brain stem, patients may also develop symptoms similar to those of Parkinson's disease.

WHAT CAN I DO TO REDUCE MY RISK OF DEVELOPING DEMENTIA?

Today, Alzheimer's disease is the seventh most common cause of death worldwide. You can't necessarily avoid getting Alzheimer's disease, but there is clear evidence that you can reduce your risk. Medical conditions such as type 2 diabetes, high blood pressure, high cholesterol and obesity are all linked to an increased probability that you will be affected, so it's important to keep these under control. People who take regular exercise, avoid smoking, and eat a healthy diet are less likely to develop the disease.

Also, anything you can do to keep your brain active will help to reduce the risk of developing dementia. Do puzzles and games, and try to stimulate your mind with conversation and reading.

HOW DEMENTIA PROGRESSES

When someone has Alzheimer's, they go on to develop much more serious problems. These typically include having difficulty with language, being unable to judge distances or dimensions, losing the ability to carry out tasks such as cooking or writing, and losing track of the day or date. In the latter stages, people may start to hallucinate. They may also become aggressive, and they will eventually lose the ability to walk, then eat. No wonder this disease is so distressing – not only for the patients themselves, but also for family members, friends and carers.

Most people do not develop Alzheimer's disease until they are over 65, although some 40,000 people in the UK are living with early-onset Alzheimer's (which develops in people aged under 65). For reasons that are not fully understood, women are roughly twice as likely to get the disease as men.

There is currently no cure for Alzheimer's disease, although certain drugs can temporarily alleviate the symptoms or slow down the progression of the disease.

The life expectancy of someone with Alzheimer's (or other types of dementia) varies considerably. After diagnosis, most people go on to live with dementia for several years, but this depends on how fit and healthy they are in other ways. Sometimes people can live for 25 years after diagnosis. Survival rates are increasing all the time, partly because people are being diagnosed earlier and are receiving better care. So if you are already quite old, there's every possibility that you could die of another cause than dementia.

There is a huge amount of scientific research being carried out around the world to find a cure for Alzheimer's disease – or at least an effective way of slowing its progress. It is also thought that some types of gene therapy may be able to prevent people from developing the illness in the first place. I anticipate that this research will make significant progress over the next few years.

CAN MEDICATION HELP WITH DEMENTIA?

Your GP may prescribe medication to control high blood pressure or cholesterol, if this is an issue for you. If your GP suspects you have multi-infarct dementia, you may be advised to take a low dose of aspirin. Dementia patients are often also prescribed an anti-depressant, as depression is a common feature of the illness.

There are also specific drugs used to treat the symptoms of dementia. Sadly, there is yet no cure for dementia, but your doctor may suggest you try these drugs. They include:

- **Acetylcholinesterase inhibitors** – acetylcholine is the chemical transmitted between nerves, and it is reduced in patients with dementia. There are strict guidelines on its use: it must be started by a specialist and its progress closely monitored. It is only used while it is deemed to be making a difference. This medication works in about half the patients who try it.
- **Memantine** – this drug reduces the chemical glutamate and seems to slow down damage to the brain cells – and therefore the progression of dementia – in some patients.

DR DAWN'S TOP TIP

Even if you are caring for someone who already has a degree of dementia, there are some simple things that you can do to keep them as independent as possible. I call them the 'Four Rs':

- **R**outine – a regular routine, and always putting things in the same place, makes it much easier to remember where things are
- **R**epetition – repeating things means they are more easily remembered
- **R**eminders – leaving notes and setting alarms to remember events helps
- **R**eminiscence – simply talking stimulates the brain.

CHAPTER 8
THE BATTLE AGAINST CANCER

We often read in the press about the need to find a cure for cancer. Of course we do, but that is somewhat simplifying the problem. Cancer is not one disease and no one cure will treat all types, however much we would like it to. Not only does cancer behave differently in different parts of the body, but any one part of the body may have different types of cancer. Currently, each one of us has a one in three chance of developing cancer, so if we are considering how we are going to live a long and healthy life, we need to consider how we can adapt our lives to minimise that risk. Currently breast, prostate, lung and bowel cancers account for just over half (53%) of all cancers in the UK. That's a sorry statistic, but the good news is that each of those cancers is linked to lifestyle. In other words, there are things we can do to help avoid developing cancer. In this chapter I will point out the things you can do to avoid certain cancers, and also the symptoms you need to look out for so that you can recognise a problem as early as possible and improve your outlook.

WHAT IS CANCER?

As I said in Chapter 2, our cells are constantly repairing themselves. Sometimes this doesn't work and the cells become abnormal and multiply out of control, forming a cancer. This can be triggered by chemicals called carcinogens (such as the chemicals found in tobacco) or workplace chemicals (such as benzene, asbestos and formaldehyde). Sometimes it happens as part of the ageing process, in which cells become damaged over time and their ability to self-repair is reduced. Cancers can also be triggered by exposure to radiation, and some are even linked to specific infections or our diet and exercise levels. There is also a genetic component to some cancers. However, it is easy to see that how we live can have a huge impact on whether or not we develop certain cancers.

If a cancer does develop, doctors need to know what type of cells there are in the cancer, how big the area of abnormality is, and how far the cells have spread. It is only when we know all these things that we can plan treatment, and also give the person an idea of their prognosis. Some cancers are easier to treat than others, but wherever the cancer, the earlier it is detected, the better the outlook. I know that sometimes fear or embarrassment means that people may delay asking for help, but I urge anyone with worrying symptoms that you fear may be cancerous to be checked out sooner rather than later. Delaying will, at best, potentially make the treatment more difficult or complex, and, at worst, could mean that doctors can only manage the symptoms of the cancer, not cure it.

WHY DO WE TALK ABOUT FIVE-YEAR SURVIVAL RATES?

Anyone who has had cancer will tell you that five years from diagnosis is a significant milestone. The longer you survive after diagnosis and treatment, the better your long-term outlook, but when doctors know exactly what type of cancer you have and how far it has spread they can predict a five-year survival figure. This is expressed as a percentage. So, a 75% five-year survival means that if we took 100 people with a particular cancer, 75 would still be alive

five years later. It gives people an idea of their chances, but it is just
a statistic. Prevention is better than cure, so let's look at some of the
most common cancers in the UK.

BREAST CANCER

Breast cancer is the most common cancer in the UK, accounting for
15% of all cancers. It is, of course, much more common in women. It
is fair to say that nothing gets a woman into my clinic room faster
than a new lump in her breast. However, the vast majority of breast
lumps are benign. Many don't require a referral and, of those that do,
nine out of ten turn out to be benign. But one in eight women will
develop breast cancer – so any breast lump needs to be checked
out.

I'm a great fan of women being breast-aware. It's your job to
know what is normal for you, so you can report any changes, and it
is my job to know whether you need further assessment. First, get
into the habit of looking at your breasts. It may feel a bit odd, but
you will notice that they are not totally symmetrical – the only
perfectly symmetrical breasts I see are silicone (and, believe me, I
have seen a lot of breasts!). It is normal for one to be slightly larger
than the other, but if one breast is changing size, then your doctor
needs to know. Take some time to look at the skin – any new
tethering (changes in appearance so the skin looks like the skin of an
orange) or dimpling should be checked out. The easiest way to
examine your own breasts is in a warm shower or bath with a soapy
hand so that you can feel your breast with the flat of your hand,
working your way around the breast and into the armpit as breast
tissue extends up into the armpit. Finally, gently squeeze both nipples
to check for any discharge. It is possible to get a milky discharge from
the nipple even when you're not breastfeeding, but any new discharge
needs to be checked out, especially if it is one-sided or blood-stained.

DR DAWN'S TOP TIP

Be breast-aware. That means looking at and feeling your breasts. Breasts can feel quite different during different times of the monthly cycle or after the menopause, so it is important that you know what is normal for you. If you notice an unusual change, report it immediately to your doctor.

WHO GETS BREAST CANCER?

Being female and getting older are the two biggest factors increasing the risk of developing breast cancer. There are around 50,000 new cases of breast cancer in the UK every year – that's almost one every ten minutes, compared to 300 a year in men. Three-quarters of all breast cancers in women occur over the age of 50, but naturally when breast cancer occurs in younger women, it hits the headlines. It can occur in young women – 1 in 20 breast cancers develop in women under the age of 35.

Having a first-degree relative (a sister, a mother or a daughter) with the disease increases your risk. For some families, we can identify genes that significantly increase the risk of developing the disease.

Women who start their periods very young or who have a late menopause are at increased risk because of their higher lifetime exposure to the female hormone oestrogen.

You can't do a lot about these things, though, so what about the things we *can* influence? Women who don't have children or who start their family late (after 30) are also at risk, but breastfeeding helps to protect against the disease.

It is also estimated that being overweight is a factor in almost one in ten cases of breast cancer, so maintaining a healthy BMI reduces your risk. Excess alcohol intake and smoking will also increase your risk, as does a high-fat diet.

DR DAWN'S TOP TIP

If you have a strong family history of breast cancer, this doesn't mean you are bound to develop the disease, but it does mean you need to consider the above list of lifestyle factors seriously and look at what you can do to counteract your genetic predisposition.

HOW DO WE SCREEN FOR BREAST CANCER?

If you are registered with an NHS GP, you will be automatically called after your 50th birthday for a mammogram. I urge you to go. You may not relish the idea of having your breasts squeezed in a machine, but the reassurance of a normal mammogram is worth it. Even if you are given bad news, early diagnosis can make all the difference to a good prognosis.

Once you are on the screening register you will be called every three years until you are 70. The screening programme is soon to be extended to include all women between 47 and 73. If you want to continue to be screened after this age, just call your local service to arrange it.

Women with a strong family history of pre-menopausal breast cancer may be offered mammogram screening at a younger age.

DR DAWN'S TOP TIP

When you are invited for a mammogram, make sure you go. If you have a strong family history of breast cancer, speak to your GP about whether you are eligible for earlier screening.

WHAT IS THE BREAST CANCER GENE?

Several genes have been identified as being associated with an increased risk of developing breast cancer. If you have a strong family history of the disease you may be offered genetic testing to look for genes including BRCA1, BRCA2 and TP53. If a woman tests positive for BRCA1, she has an 80–85% chance of developing breast cancer and will be offered a prophylactic bilateral mastectomy. This can dramatically reduce your risk – so even if your genes are against you, you can still act to protect yourself. (See also Chapter 2 for the example of Angelina Jolie.)

HOW IS BREAST CANCER DIAGNOSED?

Breast cancer is either picked up at a routine screening mammogram or is diagnosed after a woman has presented to her GP with symptoms, the most common being a painless lump.

If a woman presents with a lump that is cause for concern she will almost certainly be offered a mammogram, and possibly an ultrasound of her breasts. Ultrasound is particularly useful in premenopausal women who have more dense breast tissue. Sometimes an MRI scan will be arranged. What happens after this will depend on what the tests have shown so far. Some women will have a needle biopsy (where a sample of breast tissue is removed under local anaesthetic to be viewed under a microscope). Others may have an excision biopsy (where the entire lump is removed for analysis).

If a biopsy tests positive for cancer, then further tests will need to be done to check whether the cancer has spread. These can include blood tests, X-rays and scans.

PROSTATE CANCER

The prostate gland is a walnut-shaped gland that sits below the bladder in men. The urethra (the tube that passes urine from the bladder) runs through the middle of it. The prostate starts to enlarge any time from about the age of 50. By the age of 70, eight out of ten men will have an enlarged prostate – but that doesn't mean it is cancerous. Prostate cancer affects about one in eight men, and 40,000 men are diagnosed with prostate cancer in the UK each year, making prostate cancer the most common cancer in men. I remember being told at medical school that prostate cancer tends to be the sort of cancer you die with, not of, but it can occasionally be aggressive so it is important to recognise the symptoms and get them checked out.

WHAT ARE THE SYMPTOMS OF PROSTATE CANCER?

The symptoms of prostate cancer are the same as those of a benign (non-cancerous) enlargement of the prostate, so they are very common. While they mustn't be ignored, the good news is that they are more likely to reflect a non-cancerous problem. They include:

- **hesitancy** – the need to wait for a while before urine starts to flow
- **poor stream** – a weaker flow of urine, meaning it takes longer to empty the bladder
- **frequency** – the need to go to the toilet more frequently
- **urgency** – the need to get to the toilet more quickly
- **terminal dribbling** – a dribble of urine may trickle out after you think you have finished having a wee.

WHO GETS PROSTATE CANCER?

Like all cancers, there are some risk factors you can do nothing about, and with prostate cancer it is ageing. Most cases occur in older men. Your genetics may also play a role. If your brother or father developed prostate cancer before the age of 60 this increases your risk, and most people don't realise that having female relatives with the form of breast cancer that is linked to a faulty gene also increases a man's genetic predisposition to developing prostate cancer.

Prostate cancer is also more common in men of Afro-Caribbean descent, and less common in Asian men.

DR DAWN'S TOP TIP

Ask about your family history – it could be very relevant to your future and will help you tune in to what you need to do to stay healthy into old age.

A high-fat diet and one that is low in fruit and vegetables is thought to increase the risk of prostate cancer, and exposure to cadmium may increase the risk (cadmium is found in tobacco smoke and in the smelting and electroplating industry).

HOW IS PROSTATE CANCER DIAGNOSED?

If you develop the symptoms listed above, your doctor will want to examine your prostate. We do this by inserting a finger into your rectum to assess whether the gland is enlarged and see what it feels like. A smooth enlargement is more likely to be benign, while an enlarged prostate that feels hard or craggy is more likely to be a cancer. You will then probably be offered a blood test to measure a chemical called the prostate specific antigen (PSA), which is produced by the prostate gland. The higher the level of this chemical, the more likely you are to have a cancer. We also use the PSA blood test to assess response to treatment, as it falls with successful treatment. If the PSA is raised, you may also need a biopsy test in which a sample of prostate tissue is removed for analysis in the laboratory.

IS THERE A SCREENING TEST FOR PROSTATE CANCER?

Unfortunately, the NHS doesn't yet have a screening programme for prostate cancer in the same way as it does for breast and cervical cancer. It might seem logical to offer all men over 50 a PSA blood test, but the PSA blood test is not accurate enough. We use it in men with symptoms, in conjunction with an examination, to pick up those most likely to have a cancer, but it can sometimes be high in men without a cancer, meaning that healthy men with no symptoms could be put through invasive tests such as a biopsy for no reason. This is called a false positive result. It can also show up a false negative result – in about 15% of men with cancer it will be normal, so it is important that we look at the whole picture.

LUNG CANCER

Lung cancer remains one of the most common cancers in the UK, affecting 38,000 people every year. The majority of those affected are smokers, but one in eight cases of lung cancer occurs in people who have never smoked.

WHAT ARE THE SYMPTOMS OF LUNG CANCER?

Public Health England has been trying to raise awareness of the symptoms of lung cancer. The problem is that many of the symptoms may be ignored or attributed to a normal part of a long-term smoking habit. However, they mustn't be ignored. Sadly, if you are diagnosed with lung cancer, your prognosis remains worse than with many other cancers. That is partly because people ignore symptoms, resulting in a delay in diagnosis. Symptoms include:

- a persistent cough
- shortness of breath or wheezing
- blood-stained sputum
- fatigue and loss of energy
- chest or shoulder pain
- unexplained weight loss
- a hoarse voice
- a drooping eyelid
- clubbed fingers – if you place your thumbnails together back to back, you should see a diamond-shaped space due to the angle between the nail and the nail bed. If this is not there, we call it 'clubbing'.

DR DAWN'S TOP TIP

Some people are born with clubbed fingers. However, if your nails change it could be a sign of something serious.

WHO GETS LUNG CANCER?

Smokers, smokers, smokers! Yes, the disease does occur in non-smokers, but many of those are people who have been exposed to second-hand smoke. People who smoke up to fifteen cigarettes a day have eight times the risk of dying from lung cancer than non-smokers. Increase that to 25 or more cigarettes a day and the risk is 25 times higher. Interestingly, though, it is the length of time you smoke that is the greatest factor, so smoking 20 cigarettes a day for 20 years is riskier than smoking 40 a day for ten years, even though the total number of cigarettes smoked is the same.

There are some other factors that increase your risk: exposure to radioactive materials, nickel, chromium and asbestos. People who live in areas with high background levels of radon are also at a slightly increased risk, and bad air pollution is also thought to pose a small risk too.

Some lung cancers have a genetic link, but most lung cancers do not run in families.

HOW IS LUNG CANCER DIAGNOSED?

The first test that your doctor will arrange if they suspect lung cancer is a chest X-ray. After this you may need further scans or a bronchoscopy (a look into the lungs with a specially designed telescope).

BOWEL CANCER

Bowel cancer is also called colon cancer or colorectal cancer. It is the third most common cancer in the UK, affecting around 40,000 people every year.

WHAT ARE THE SYMPTOMS OF COLON CANCER?

In the early stages, bowel cancer may have no symptoms at all. When symptoms develop they can include:

- bleeding from the rectum or blood in your stools
- abdominal pain
- a change in bowel habits, which could be towards constipation or diarrhoea
- unexplained weight loss
- a lump in the abdomen
- symptoms of anaemia as a result of blood loss – a pale look, shortness of breath on minimal exertion, fatigue and chest pain.

DR DAWN'S TOP TIP

Don't ignore the symptoms above – the chances are they will be nothing serious. For example, bleeding from the back passage is most likely to be caused by haemorrhoids, but it must never be ignored.

WHO GETS COLON CANCER?

Four-fifths of bowel cancers occur in the over-60s. About 5% are due to inherited conditions such as familial adenomatous polyposis (FAP) or Lynch syndrome. Other risk factors include having other conditions including:

- polyps
- Crohn's disease and ulcerative colitis
- diabetes
- testicular cancer
- womb cancer
- lymphoma.

It's not just down to the luck of the draw. Drinking too much alcohol and eating a diet high in red and processed meat increases your risk of developing the disease. A high-fibre diet seems to protect against this cancer, so make sure you eat at least five portions of fruit and vegetables every day. Eating fish also probably reduces the risk, as does a calcium-rich diet. And just in case you need yet another reason to watch your weight, being obese also increases the risk of developing bowel cancer.

Take regular exercise and don't smoke, as this will reduce your risk. Studies have also shown that taking a daily low-dose aspirin protects against colon cancer – but discuss this with your doctor first, as aspirin can cause side-effects which may mean it is not appropriate for you.

Hormone replacement therapy and the combined contraceptive pill may also be protective.

HOW IS COLON CANCER DIAGNOSED?

If your GP suspects colon cancer, they will refer you urgently for a colonoscopy. If there is anything suspicious to be seen on the colonoscopy, the specialist will take biopsies to be analysed under a microscope. If cancer is confirmed, then you will have further tests to see if the cancer has spread.

CAN I BE SCREENED FOR COLON CANCER?

If you are registered with an NHS GP in England and are aged between 60 and 69, you will be offered bowel screening in the form of a testing kit that you will be sent in the post. The screening programme includes people up to 74 in Scotland and Wales and starts at 50 in Wales. There are plans to extend the screening programme so that everyone in the UK will be offered the test between the ages of 50 and 74. The test involves smearing a small sample of your poo onto a test card, which you then send back to be analysed in the laboratory for microscopic traces of blood. It may not sound much like fun but it is a simple test that could save your life. If the sample tests positive for blood, you will be offered a colonoscopy. There are plans to include a one-off sigmoidoscopy (a look into the bowel using a special camera) for everyone over 55.

You may also be screened if:

- you have had bowel cancer before
- you have had polyps
- you have FAP or Lynch syndrome
- you have several relatives with bowel cancer
- you have Crohn's disease or ulcerative colitis.

DR DAWN'S TOP TIP

Less than half of bowel screening test kits are returned. Don't let yours be one of them. It's a simple, free and painless test which could save your life! (I have several patients who are proof of that fact.)

MELANOMA

Melanoma is the least common, but most serious, form of skin cancer, affecting around 9,000 people in the UK each year, many of them young adults. Melanoma is the second most common cancer in people aged 15 to 34. Its incidence has almost doubled in the UK in the past couple of decades, probably related to the increase in foreign travel and sun exposure.

WHAT ARE THE SYMPTOMS OF MELANOMA?

A melanoma can develop in normal skin or in an existing mole. The signs to look for are easiest to remember as A, B, C, D, E:

- **A**symmetry – a melanoma is usually irregular, not symmetrical
- **B**order – the edges of a melanoma are usually ragged or blurred
- **C**olour – the colour of a melanoma is uneven, with different pigments
- **D**iameter – a melanoma is often greater than 6 mm in diameter, although if a mole is changing don't ignore it just because it isn't this big
- **E**volving – if a mole is changing in any way in terms of A, B, C or D, or if it starts to itch or bleed or crust over, it must be checked urgently.

WHO GETS MELANOMA?

At least 60% of melanomas are related to UV light exposure, either from the sun or from sunbeds. People with fair skin are most at risk. Darker skins have more pigment, which acts as a mild natural sun protection factor. This shouldn't be relied on, though – it probably only amounts to sun protection factor (SPF) 2–4, and we should be using at least SPF 15. Children's skin is most vulnerable: just one episode of sunburn as a child can double a child's risk of developing a skin cancer (of which melanoma is just one) in adulthood.

Other risk factors include:

- a family history – if a close blood relative has melanoma, your risk is doubled and you need to protect your skin
- having more than 100 existing moles on your body
- having a weak immune system – if you are taking immunosuppressant drugs or are HIV-positive then you have an increased risk.

DR DAWN'S TOP TIP

Don't use sunbeds, especially if you have red hair or are under 20, as that makes you more susceptible to the damage caused by UV rays in sunbeds. It's just not worth it. There are excellent tans available out of a bottle these days, so use them instead.

HOW IS MELANOMA DIAGNOSED?

If your doctor is concerned that you may have a melanoma, they will arrange for the entire mole to be surgically removed immediately. The sample will be checked in the laboratory to ensure it has all been removed.

KIDNEY CANCER

In the UK 11,900 people develop kidney cancer each year. There are several types of kidney cancer. The most common type develops in the tubules of the kidneys and is called renal cell cancer.

WHAT ARE THE SYMPTOMS OF KIDNEY CANCER?

The most common initial symptom is blood in the urine. This is called haematuria. While most cases of haematuria will be caused by something far less worrying, such as an infection, blood in the urine must never be ignored.

DR DAWN'S TOP TIP

Check the colour of your urine. If there is a lot of blood present, it will look red and will be obvious, but smaller amounts may just tinge the urine pink. This should be checked out. Ask yourself one question first, though – have you been eating beetroot? Beetroot will colour your urine pink!
   Other symptoms include:
* pain in your side or back
* night sweats
* fatigue
* weight loss
* signs of anaemia.

WHO GETS KIDNEY CANCER?

Many people who develop kidney cancer just seem to be unlucky – it happens for no obvious reason. I wanted to include it here because there *are* some things we can do to reduce our risk, and they may not seem that obvious. Being overweight and smoking, for example, both increase the risk of kidney cancer. People who work with organic solvents, cadmium and asbestos are also at increased risk. Most people who develop kidney cancer do so over the age of 60 and in fact it is uncommon under the age of 50.

HOW IS KIDNEY CANCER DIAGNOSED?

Most kidney cancers are actually diagnosed on a scan which may have been arranged for other reasons.

HEAD AND NECK CANCERS

While the incidence of many cancers is reducing, sadly, the incidence of head and neck cancers is increasing. Experts predict that numbers could increase by a third in the next 20 years.

WHAT ARE THE SYMPTOMS OF HEAD AND NECK CANCER?

The signs to look out for include:

• red or white patches in the mouth
• a lump on the lip or in the mouth or neck
• pain when chewing or swallowing
• a change in your voice
• unusual bleeding or numbness in the mouth or throat.

DR DAWN'S TOP TIP

Have regular dental check-ups – dentists are trained to look for the early signs of head and neck cancer as part of a routine check-up.

WHO GETS HEAD AND NECK CANCER?

Smoking and alcohol are the real problems. They both increase the risk, but smoking and drinking excessively increases the risk even more. Chewing tobacco is also a risk, as is poor dental hygiene, but the good news is that a healthy, well-balanced diet seems to protect against the disease.

HOW IS HEAD AND NECK CANCER DIAGNOSED?

If head and neck cancer is suspected, your doctor or dentist will arrange for a small sample of tissue (a biopsy) to be sent to the laboratory to be assessed under a microscope.

BRAIN CANCER

Brain tumours can strike at any age. Sometimes they affect young children, but most brain tumours occur in people aged over 50. About 5,000 people in the UK are diagnosed each year with a primary brain tumour, and many more have a secondary brain tumour, which has spread from cancer in another site, such as the lung or breast.

WHAT ARE THE SYMPTOMS OF A BRAIN TUMOUR?

This depends largely on where the tumour is in the brain, but symptoms include:

- persistent severe headaches
- fits
- vomiting

- drowsiness
- personality changes
- signs of a stroke (such as slurred speech, visual problems, drooping of one side of the face, or weakness in the limbs).

WHO GETS BRAIN TUMOURS?

People with a close relative who has had a brain tumour may have a slightly increased risk, and there are some tumours that are linked to genetic conditions such as neurofibromatosis (a condition made famous by the Elephant Man, Joseph Merrick). Exposure to radiation increases the risk of developing a brain tumour.

I am often asked about the possible risks associated with mobile phone use. The theory is that radiofrequency emitted by mobile phones could heat cells and potentially damage them. Studies are under way to evaluate this further, but there is currently no evidence that mobile phone use is in any way linked to the later development of brain tumours. (That said, when my children were younger I used to ask them not to charge their phones by their beds at night. This was more to do with helping them get an undisturbed night's sleep rather than spending half the night on social media sites!)

HOW ARE BRAIN TUMOURS DIAGNOSED?

Most brain tumours are diagnosed following a CT or an MRI scan.

BLADDER CANCER

About 10,000 people get bladder cancer each year in the UK. Around 80% of these are superficial tumours that are easily treated. The other 20% are more invasive tumours, and more likely to spread, making them less likely to be cured.

WHAT ARE THE SYMPTOMS OF BLADDER CANCER?

Just like kidney cancer, the most common symptom is blood in the urine, so always get this symptom checked out. Symptoms may also mirror those of a urinary infection – needing to pass urine more frequently, and burning or stinging while passing urine.

WHO GETS BLADDER CANCER?

As with all cancers, there are some risk factors we can do little about, such as getting older (bladder cancer is rare in people under 40), being male (bladder cancer is three times more common in men than in women), or being Caucasian.

But there are other things that we definitely can do something about. Few people realise that smoking is a significant risk factor for bladder cancer, and so is exposure to certain workplace chemicals, such as those used in the rubber and dye industry. Thankfully, most of these are now banned in the UK but as bladder cancer can develop decades after exposure, it is important to bear that association in mind. Previous chemotherapy or radiotherapy may also increase the risk, as does previous schistosomiasis (also called bilharzia) infection. This is a bladder infection caused by a parasitic worm found in tropical and subtropical fresh waters, most commonly in Africa.

More recently we have seen evidence of damage to the bladder lining in people who regularly use the recreational drug ketamine. The symptoms mimic those of bladder cancer. Doctors have not yet seen evidence that using the drug could lead to bladder cancer, but it's a possibility – and certainly a good enough reason to give the drug a miss.

HOW IS BLADDER CANCER DIAGNOSED?

Most cases of bladder cancer will be diagnosed by a cystoscopy. This is where we use a special telescope to look directly into the bladder. Biopsies can be taken from any areas of the bladder wall that look suspicious.

PANCREATIC CANCER

Just over 9,500 people get pancreatic cancer each year. That's 3% of all the cancers in the UK.

WHAT ARE THE SYMPTOMS OF PANCREATIC CANCER?

Unfortunately, pancreatic cancer generally has a poor prognosis, and this is largely because it often presents late – in the early stages, there may be no symptoms. It is only when the tumour has grown large enough to cause a blockage of the bile duct that people become jaundiced, their urine becomes very dark, and their stools may be very pale, loose and floaty. Generalised itching may also be a symptom. As the tumour progresses, there may also be abdominal or back pain and unexplained weight loss. Rarely, pancreatic cancer presents with type 2 diabetes.

DR DAWN'S TOP TIP

I was at a conference recently at which we were discussing pancreatic cancer. One specialist proposed that if someone with a healthy BMI were diagnosed with type 2 diabetes, doctors should arrange an ultrasound scan to exclude pancreatic cancer. This is not routinely done, but we have adopted this policy in my practice. If you are diagnosed with type 2 diabetes but are a healthy BMI, ask your GP about an ultrasound scan. If pancreatic cancer is picked up early, the outlook is greatly improved.

WHO GETS PANCREATIC CANCER?

Most people who get pancreatic cancer are over 60, and most have a number of lifestyle factors that significantly increase the risk. These include obesity, smoking, excess alcohol consumption, and a high-fat diet with lots of red meat. There does also seem to be an increased risk in people exposed to some pesticides, dyes and chemicals used in the metal refining industry.

Most pancreatic cancers do not have a genetic link, but it is thought that about one in ten is due to the inheritance of an abnormal gene.

HOW IS PANCREATIC CANCER DIAGNOSED?

If your doctor is concerned about the possibility of pancreatic cancer, they will arrange an ultrasound scan of your abdomen in the first instance.

LEUKAEMIA

Leukaemia is cancer of the blood, and there are several different forms.

WHAT ARE THE SYMPTOMS OF LEUKAEMIA?

It depends which cells in the blood are affected. If the red cells are affected, leukaemia may present with symptoms of anaemia. If it is the cells that help the blood to clot that are involved, then it will be problems with bleeding – bleeding gums are a common presentation. And if the problem is to do with the white cells, then recurrent or unusual infections may occur. There could be any combination of these symptoms too.

WHO GETS LEUKAEMIA?

It is thought that leukaemia starts with just one cell becoming abnormal, but why this should happen is not always clear. Some factors seem to increase the risk, such as exposure to radiation, previous chemotherapy, or exposure to chemicals such as benzene. There is occasionally a genetic link – people with Down's syndrome, for example, have an increased risk of developing leukaemia.

HOW IS LEUKAEMIA DIAGNOSED?

A blood test may show up abnormalities that suggest leukaemia, and the diagnosis is then confirmed with a bone marrow test. This involves a small needle being inserted into the pelvic bone (or sometimes the breast bone) under local anaesthetic so that a sample of bone marrow can be taken for analysis in the laboratory.

UTERINE CANCER

You may never even have thought about the prospect of cancer of the womb – it isn't common so, unlike breast cancer, you may not know anyone who has suffered from the condition. Uterine cancer (also known as endometrial cancer) affects around 7,500 women in the UK each year, mostly women over 50. The more exposure to oestrogen a woman has during her lifetime, the greater her risk of developing the condition. So the earlier you start your periods and the later you go through the menopause, the greater your risk. Being overweight will also increase your chance of developing uterine cancer, since fat cells generate oestrogen. Women who do not have children are also at risk. There is a small increased risk in diabetics, those taking tamoxifen (a breast cancer drug) and women with polycystic ovary syndrome. Interestingly, there are fewer cases of uterine cancer in Eastern countries and some experts think that a Western diet high in fat may also pose a risk.

WHAT ARE THE SYMPTOMS OF UTERINE CANCER?

The most common symptom of uterine cancer is bleeding after going through the menopause, so no post-menopausal bleed should be ignored. I have lost count of the number of endometrial biopsy tests I have done to investigate post-menopausal bleeding. Thankfully, I can count the cases of uterine cancer on the fingers of one hand, so don't panic if you start bleeding after going through the change – but don't ignore it either.

Other symptoms include bleeding after sex or between periods, pain during or after sex, and an unexplained vaginal discharge.

HOW IS UTERINE CANCER DIAGNOSED?

If your doctor wants to rule out the possibility of uterine cancer, they will arrange for you to have an endometrial biopsy test. This involves passing a small straw-like device through the neck of your womb to collect some cells using gentle suction. These cells are then analysed under a microscope to look for abnormalities. You will also have an ultrasound test to look at the thickness of the womb lining – this may be done with a probe on the lower abdomen or via the vagina, but is completely painless. It may also be suggested that you have a hysteroscopy, in which a small telescope is inserted into the womb to look at the lining directly. If any areas look abnormal samples of tissue can be removed for further analysis.

As with all cancers, it is important to establish the spread of the disease before deciding on a treatment plan. If you are faced with a diagnosis, you will then be given further tests, including blood tests, X-rays and scans to find out how far the cancer has spread.

OESOPHAGEAL CANCER

There are two types of oesophageal cancer, both of which are thankfully not common, but they are becoming significantly more frequent in the UK so it is important that we cover them in this chapter. The most common form starts in the mucous glands lining the oesophagus. This is called adenocarcinoma. It tends to form in the lower third of the oesophagus, and accounts for 60% of all cases of carcinoma of the oesophagus. The other 40% of cases start in the squamous cells lining the oesophagus, and this type of cancer is called squamous cell carcinoma.

WHAT ARE THE SYMPTOMS OF OESOPHAGEAL CANCER?

In the early stages you may not have any symptoms but as the cancer grows you are likely to find it difficult to swallow food. Initially this will only happen with very solid food, but if the cancer is left untreated it will occur with softer foods and even ultimately liquids. You are likely to lose weight without trying. You may be sick frequently, and the vomit may contain blood. Some people develop a cough or a hoarse voice.

WHO GETS OESOPHAGEAL CANCER?

There is no one specific cause for oesophageal cancer, but we know that several factors increase the risk of it developing. These include

- age – most cases occur in over-55s
- gender – it is more common in men than in women

- geography – oesophageal cancer is more common in China than it is in the UK, although we don't yet know why
- alcohol – heavy drinkers and especially heavy spirit drinkers are most at risk
- smoking – the more you smoke, the greater your risk
- gastro-oesophageal reflux disease (GORD) – long-term exposure of the oesophagus to acid increases the risk
- flushing – people who flush when they drink alcohol lack an enzyme called aldehyde dehydrogenase two (ALDH2). One study[1] has made a link between this and developing oesophageal cancer.

DR DAWN'S TOP TIP

Watch your alcohol intake, especially if you flush when you drink or suffer from indigestion the morning after – your body could be trying to tell you something!

HOW IS OESOPHAGEAL CANCER DIAGNOSED?

The initial diagnosis is likely to be made by endoscopy. The doctor will biopsy any suspicious-looking areas so that they can be examined under the microscope. If a cancer is confirmed on biopsy, the specialists will then arrange for various scans and other tests to check whether the cancer has spread.

OVARIAN CANCER

It often surprises women when they hear that ovarian cancer is more common than cervical cancer. It is the fifth most common cancer in women in the UK. There are three different types of ovarian cancer, but by far the most common form (accounting for

90% of all ovarian cancers) is epithelial ovarian cancer, in which the cancer forms in the cells surrounding the ovary. Other forms arise from the cells that make eggs (germ cell ovarian cancer) or the cells that produce hormones (stromal ovarian cancer)

WHAT ARE THE SYMPTOMS OF OVARIAN CANCER?

Sadly, ovarian cancer has been called 'the silent killer' because the early symptoms may be vague and can be attributed to other much more common conditions, typically irritable bowel syndrome. If you have a family history of ovarian cancer it is important that you take note of the presenting symptoms and report them to your GP. Constant pain in the pelvis and persistent bloating should not be ignored – it is the persistence that is key. We all get bloated from time to time, but if it doesn't settle (and particularly if it is associated with a feeling of being full very quickly), it should be checked out.

Ovarian cancer may also make your tummy look distended. It can cause you to lose weight. You may need to pass water more frequently or you may be constipated. You may also experience pain in the lower abdomen or in your back.

WHAT CAUSES EPITHELIAL OVARIAN CANCER?

There is no one specific cause, but most cases occur after the menopause so increasing age is a definite risk factor. Anything that increases oestrogen exposure will also increase the risk – so being overweight or obese, not having children, or having a late menopause are all risk factors for ovarian cancer.

In a minority of cases (about one in ten) there is a genetic component – carriers of the BRCA1 and BRCA2 genes are at increased risk. If you have a strong family history of breast and ovarian cancer at a young age, it is worth talking to your GP about being tested for these genes. You will need to have counselling because you will have to make some major decisions if your test is positive.

WHY DOESN'T THE NHS SCREEN FOR OVARIAN CANCER LIKE IT DOES FOR BREAST AND CERVICAL CANCER?

For a screening test to be useful, it must be sensitive enough to pick up as many cases as possible – and it mustn't flag up too many false positives. The smear test (looking for precancerous cells on the cervix) and the mammogram for breast cancer fulfil these criteria well. Work is being done on a screening test, which could include a blood test looking for a protein called CA-125 which is raised in ovarian cancer, and an ultrasound. The outlook for women with ovarian cancer would be massively improved if doctors could find a way of detecting the disease earlier, but at the moment the tests aren't specific enough to use on all women: there would be too many false positives, and some women would end up undergoing unnecessary surgery.

That said, women who have two or more close relatives who have had premenopausal breast cancer or ovarian cancer may be offered the tests that are currently available, as their risk is significantly higher than that of the general population.

STOMACH CANCER

Stomach cancer is relatively uncommon but, as with all cancers, the sooner it is detected, the better the outlook.

WHAT ARE THE SYMPTOMS OF STOMACH CANCER?

The symptoms of stomach cancer may include feeling full very quickly, feeling sick or losing your appetite, discomfort in the upper abdomen, or having persistent indigestion. Occasionally, if the cancer is starting to cause bleeding, your stools may look black and tarry.

WHO GETS STOMACH CANCER?

There are a number of factors that increase your risk. These include:

* gender – men are twice as likely as women to develop stomach cancer
* age – most cases occur in the over-55s
* smoking – people who smoke are twice as likely to develop stomach cancer
* *helicobacter pylori* infection – a bacteria that lives in the stomach and causes indigestion
* stomach ulcers
* family history – if you have a close relative with stomach cancer, this doubles your risk
* diet – a diet rich in pickled vegetables, salt and smoked meats increases your risk
* blood type A – being blood type A is associated with an increased risk
* another cancer – having another cancer, including bowel, prostate, bladder, testicle, breast, ovarian or cervical cancer, can also increase your risk.

HOW IS STOMACH CANCER DIAGNOSED?

Your doctor will arrange an endoscopy. If they suspect cancer, then biopsies will be taken at the time for analysis in the laboratory. You may also have an ultrasound test and a barium swallow. If these confirm cancer, then your doctor will arrange further tests, which will probably include a CT or MRI scan to assess whether the cancer has spread outside the stomach, as this will affect the treatment you will need.

LIVER CANCER

Cancer that starts in the liver is rare. It is much more common for a cancer elsewhere in the body to spread to the liver. This is called secondary liver cancer. Around 5,400 people in the UK get primary liver cancer each year. It tends to occur in people over 70 and is more common in men. Unfortunately it is one of the cancers that is on the rise in the UK and that is thought to be because of increased alcohol consumption.

WHAT ARE THE SYMPTOMS OF LIVER CANCER?

Liver cancer can present as:

- unexplained weight loss
- abdominal pain or swelling
- fluid retention
- jaundice
- sweats
- itching.

DR DAWN'S TOP TIP

I have referred to unexplained weight loss in relation to a few cancers, so I will explain what I mean by this. Most people's weight fluctuates by a few pounds here and there, but anyone who loses more than 10% of their body weight without trying to do so should have a medical check up. If you normally weigh around ten stone and have lost a stone, you need to know why – your doctor will look into it for you. It may be something as simple as a subtle change in your lifestyle or an overactive thyroid, but significant unexplained weight loss should never be ignored.

WHO GETS LIVER CANCER?

People who have existing liver problems such as cirrhosis, non-alcoholic fatty liver, primary biliary cirrhosis, a genetic condition called hemochromatosis, or hepatitis are at increased risk of developing liver cancer. And yes, you guessed it, being overweight, smoking and drinking to excess are all risk factors for developing the disease.

HOW IS LIVER CANCER DIAGNOSED?

The diagnosis is usually made following scans and a biopsy.

DR DAWN'S TOP TIP

If you have one of the known existing liver diseases that predisposes you to liver cancer, talk to your GP about regular surveillance scans so that if you should develop the disease it is picked up early.

THYROID CANCER

Thyroid cancer is most often found in people in their forties. It is more common in women.

WHAT ARE THE SYMPTOMS OF THYROID CANCER?

The common symptoms include:

• a lump in the neck (although only 1 in 20 lumps in the neck turns out to be cancer)
• persistent hoarseness lasting more than three weeks
• a sore throat lasting more than three weeks
• difficulty swallowing.

WHO GETS THYROID CANCER?

If you have existing thyroiditis or a family history of thyroid disease, your risk is increased, but an under- or overactive thyroid is not linked to thyroid cancer. A rare inherited condition called familial adenomatous polyposis (FAP), which increases the risk of bowel cancer, also increases the risk of thyroid cancer, as does acromegaly (gigantism) and being obese.

HOW IS THYROID CANCER DIAGNOSED?

Most thyroid cancers are diagnosed with a scan and biopsy test.

CERVICAL CANCER

Cervical cancer is a largely preventable disease. In 99% of cases, infection with the human papilloma virus (HPV) is to blame. Now that we have effective vaccination against this virus, and as long as women attend smear tests (also known as cervical screening) when called, we should be able to all but eradicate the disease. Today around 1,000 women die each year of cervical cancer. This disease is most common in women in their thirties and forties, so anything that can be done to reduce that number has to be a priority. Below, I look at the screening programme in the UK to persuade you of its value.

WHAT ARE THE SYMPTOMS OF CERVICAL CANCER?

There may be no symptoms at all in the early stages, which is why it is so important that women attend smear tests, so that precancerous changes can be picked up and dealt with. If symptoms do develop they may include abnormal bleeding, such as bleeding after sex, between periods, or after the menopause. These symptoms are relatively common and usually due to much less serious problems, but they should never be ignored.

WHO GETS CERVICAL CANCER?

Virtually all sexually active women will have been exposed to HPV, but some women don't clear the virus effectively – and they are at risk of developing cervical cancer. Women who smoke, and anyone with a suppressed immune system (such as women with AIDS, or taking immune suppressant medication) are more at risk. There has been a slight increase in risk in women taking the combined oral contraceptive pill for more than eight years.

There are over 100 different types of HPV. Some cause warts and verrucas, while others are responsible for changes in the cervix that can lead to cervical cancer. In fact, it is thought that 99% of cases of cervical cancer are caused by infection with high-risk types of HPV, known as types 16 and 18. For most women, they cause no problems at all. There are no symptoms associated with the infection, and our immune system simply clears the virus over time. In some cases, however, the infection persists, causing precancerous cells in the cervix.

There is now a vaccine against the high-risk strains of HPV. This is offered to all girls in the UK aged 12–13. It is given as separate injections several months apart. It is offered to girls before they become sexually active, therefore preventing them being infected with the virus.

DR DAWN'S TOP TIP

I believe that cervical cancer is an almost totally preventable disease. If you or someone you love is offered a vaccine or a smear test, make sure it is accepted – it could save a life.

WHAT ABOUT CERVICAL SCREENING?

It's a common misconception that when we call women for a cervical smear, it is to test for cervical cancer. In fact, the smear test is looking for changes in cells in the cervix that, if left unchecked, could over a period of years become cancerous. That's why it is so important to attend for a smear when called – the smear test is designed to help prevent cancer, not diagnose it.

WHAT DOES A SMEAR TEST INVOLVE?

If you are registered with an NHS GP and are eligible for a smear test (see below), you will routinely be called to see the nurse in your practice. You will be asked to lie on your back on an examination couch, place your feet together, bring your feet up to your bottom and allow your knees to fall apart. It's not the most glamorous or dignified of positions but, rest assured, it is all in a day's work for medical staff. The more relaxed you can be about it, the easier it will be for the nurse or GP to take the smear – and the more comfortable it will be for you. A small instrument called a speculum will be placed into the vagina. The speculum is then opened like the beak of a duck so that the cervix can be seen.

A small plastic brush is used to sweep around the cervix (which you shouldn't be able to feel at all) and the cells that are collected are put into a pot containing a special fluid before being sent to a laboratory for analysis under a microscope. When you have your smear, check with the nurse how long it will be before you get the results – it is usually a few weeks.

WHO CAN HAVE A SMEAR TEST?

If you are registered with an NHS GP you will automatically be called for your first smear after your 25th birthday if you live in England or Northern Ireland. It will be after your 20th birthday if you live in Wales or Scotland. As long as everything is normal, you will be called every three years until your 49th birthday. After that your smears will be less frequent as you have a lower risk of abnormalities developing. After the age of 50, you will be called every five years until the age of 65. After that you will not be routinely called unless previous smears have been abnormal.

WHY DON'T WOMEN UNDER 25 GET CALLED IN ENGLAND AND NORTHERN IRELAND FOR SMEAR TESTS?

We used to screen women in England and Northern Ireland from the age of 20, and the decision to increase the age for the first smear to 25 was based on the evidence that cervical cancer is (thankfully) extremely rare under the age of 25, whereas abnormal results are relatively common in this age group. The vast majority of the abnormalities found in such young women revert to normal without the need for any treatment, but of course cause a lot of anxiety along the way.

That said, it is important that sexually active women under the age of 25 know that they should report symptoms such as abnormal bleeding between periods or after sex, and any unexplained vaginal bleeding. The vast majority of these cases won't be cancer at all, but symptoms like this should be checked out.

DO I HAVE TO HAVE A SMEAR TEST IF I HAVE NEVER HAD SEX?

By far and away the most significant risk factor for developing cervical cancer is infection with the human papilloma virus, which is spread by sexual contact. However, there are other, less common, types of cervical cancer, so it is important you have regular smear tests.

DO I HAVE TO HAVE A SMEAR TEST IF I AM GAY?

For the same reason as above, it is a good idea to go for your smear test when you are called. Even if you are gay and you have never had a heterosexual relationship, HPV can be spread between same-sex couples, so please attend regular smear tests.

DO I HAVE TO HAVE A SMEAR TEST IF I HAVE HAD A HYSTERECTOMY?

Most hysterectomies involve removing the whole of the womb, including the cervix, but do check with your doctor – occasionally the neck of the womb (the cervix) is left. This is called a subtotal hysterectomy. If you have had this type of hysterectomy you will need to continue having regular smears. If you have had a hysterectomy to remove a cancer you will need to attend for what is called a vault smear. This is the same as a cervical smear, but cells are taken from the top of the vagina to check that no cancerous cells have been left in place.

CAN I HAVE A SMEAR WHEN I AM HAVING A PERIOD?

The best time to have a smear is mid-cycle, so if your appointment comes through for a time when you think you will be bleeding it is best to reschedule it. The main reason for this is that the blood may mean that not enough cells are collected and you would need to have the test repeated.

WHAT DO THE RESULTS OF A SMEAR TEST MEAN?

Smear tests will be reported in one of three ways – as normal, inadequate or abnormal:

- **Normal** – Nine out of ten smears are reported as normal. If this is you, you will simply be called again in three or five years, depending on your age. Of course, you should remember that no test is 100% accurate, so if you should develop symptoms before your next test is due, make sure you report them to your doctor.
- **Inadequate** – This simply means that not enough cells were collected and you will be asked to return for a repeat test. If you have three consecutive inadequate tests, you will be referred for a colposcopy (see below).
- **Abnormal** – Only about 1 in 20 smears is reported as abnormal, and there are varying degrees of abnormality, from what is described as a borderline case to invasive disease. It is important to remember that the vast majority of abnormal smears are *not* cancerous, and nine out of ten significant changes known as dyskaryosis actually revert to normal without the need for treatment. Most abnormal smear results will simply mean that you are asked to attend for a repeat smear at a shorter

time interval to check that the changes are resolving. If the abnormalities are more severe, or if changes don't improve on their own, you will be referred for a colposcopy.

WHAT IS A COLPOSCOPY?

A colposcopy is a more detailed look at the cervix. It is usually done in outpatients by a trained doctor or nurse. You will be asked to lie on an examination couch and your feet will be put into stirrups. A speculum is used, just as in a normal smear test, but instead of looking directly at the cervix, the doctor or nurse uses a special telescope called a colposcope. This doesn't go inside you but is placed between your legs. A special liquid is used to paint the cervix, which helps to highlight any abnormal cells, but you won't feel that, then a small sample of tissue is taken from the cervix for in-depth analysis in the laboratory. The whole thing should only take about 15 minutes, and you will be given a follow-up appointment to decide whether any further treatment is required once the results are available.

This chapter has not given an exhaustive list of every form of cancer. That would make a medical textbook all on its own, but I hope I have covered the more common cancers in the UK and given you an idea of how you can try to reduce your chances of developing them.

DR DAWN'S TOP TIP

There is a genetic component to many cancers (and to many other illnesses), so spend some time looking into your family's medical history. If you come across a cancer not mentioned in this chapter, look it up. You can't change your genes but there will almost certainly be something you can change in your lifestyle to try to counter any genetic risk.

CHAPTER 9
YOUR BEST SHOT

In this book I have tried to show you how you can influence how long and how well you live. It is not intended to be a fully comprehensive medical textbook, and I can't cover every single medical condition that may affect your longevity in a book like this, but I think it is important to include some of the infections that have historically been major killers – and that still could be. Prior to the introduction of widespread vaccinations, measles caused an estimated 2.6 million deaths each year. Today in the UK a fatality from measles makes newspaper headlines because it is so rare, but measles remains one of the leading causes of death in children globally. All children and adults registered with an NHS GP in the UK are offered a comprehensive vaccination schedule to protect them against many of the diseases that used to kill far too many people prematurely.

Thousands of articles have been written about the potential risks of vaccination. Andrew Wakefield first questioned a possible link between the MMR (measles, mumps and rubella) vaccine and autism, and suggested that more research needed to be done. That work has now been done, and no link has been proven. I am confident enough about the safety of the vaccine that all three of my children had both doses of the MMR, and I would do the same today. It is, of course, right that there are reporting systems in place so that if any safety issues arise, they are picked up quickly.

All vaccines in the UK have to be passed by the Joint

Committee on Vaccination and Immunisation. This is an independent advisory committee comprising specialists and including lay members of the public, which looks at all the research before passing a vaccination as safe. So the vaccines that are offered in the UK are safe – but the diseases they protect against are not. They kill and maim people. Believe me, you only have to meet one baby born congenitally deaf and mute as a result of a pregnant woman having contracted rubella, or see a young adult living with severe learning difficulties as a result of measles encephalitis, to be convinced of the benefit of our vaccination schedule. All three of my children had all their vaccinations, and I would do the same if I had young children today. I encourage my patients to attend for vaccinations when they are called, and I will do the same myself. There is no doubt in my mind that, if we want to live a long and fulfilled life, we need to take advantage of all the protection we can. However, if you are concerned about whether or not your child should have any vaccine, please discuss this with your GP.

THE IMMUNISATION SCHEDULE IN THE UK

If you and your family are registered with an NHS GP, you will automatically be sent appointments for these vaccinations. If you miss an appointment or can't make one, simply call your surgery and they will reschedule for you.

- **2 months**
  5-in-1 vaccine
  Pneumococcal vaccine
  Rotavirus vaccine
  Meningitis B vaccine

- **3 months**
  5-in-1 vaccine
  Rotavirus vaccine
  Meningitis C vaccine
- **4 months**
  5-in-1 vaccine
  Pneumococcal vaccine
  Meningitis B vaccine
- **12 months**
  Meningitis B vaccine (this is often given at the same time as the vaccines below)
- **12–13 months**
  Hib/Men. C booster
  Pneumococcal vaccine
  MMR vaccine
- **2–7 years**
  Influenza vaccine (flu) – annual dose
- **3 years, 4 months**
  4-in-1 (DTaP/IPV) preschool booster
  MMR (2nd dose)
- **12–13 years (girls only)**
  HPV vaccine
- **14 years**
  3-in-1 teenage booster (diphtheria, tetanus and polio)
  Men. ACWY vaccine
- **65 years**
  Pneumococcal vaccine
- **65 and over**
  Flu vaccine (every year)
- **70 years (and 78- and 79-year-olds as catch-up)**
  Shingles vaccine

THE VACCINATIONS

5-IN-1 VACCINE

The 5-in-1 vaccine is also sometimes referred to as the DTaP/IPV/
Hib vaccine. It is given as a single injection, usually into a baby's thigh.
It protects against diphtheria, tetanus, whooping cough (pertussis),
polio and haemophilus influenza type b (Hib). It may cause your
baby to be a little irritable that evening, and there may be some
redness around the injection site. There is no active ingredient in the
vaccine so it is safe.

PNEUMOCOCCAL VACCINE

This is also given as an injection and may cause a mild fever, redness
or hardness at the injection site.

ROTAVIRUS VACCINE

This is given by liquid dropper directly into the mouth. The vaccine
contains a weakened form of the virus, which is not strong enough
to cause infection but is strong enough to trigger the immune
system to develop immunity to future rotavirus infections. Since its
introduction, there has been a 70% fall in cases of rotavirus, a
common cause of diarrhoea and sickness.

MENINGITIS B VACCINE

This is also given by injection. It is made from three proteins found
on the surface of the meningitis B bacteria. It has no active
ingredient, so it cannot cause meningitis. It may cause a fever 24
hours after vaccination, and some redness at the injection site. Your
baby may also be slightly irritable for a short period.

MENINGITIS C VACCINE

This is made using part of the surface of the meningitis C vaccine so again is very safe. It may cause redness at the site of infection, and fever, and occasionally babies vomit after the injection. It was introduced in 1999. Amazingly, meningitis C has been virtually eradicated from the UK as a result!

HIB/MEN. C BOOSTER

This is an inactivated vaccine designed to boost immunity to these infections in future.

MMR VACCINE

This vaccine contains weakened versions of the viruses that cause measles, mumps and rubella. Thousands of articles have been written about a possible link between this vaccine and autism but, despite multiple research projects, no link has ever been proven. Autism is a disorder of communication and socialisation, and it starts to become obvious when your child begins to speak and communicate – which is also when they are given the vaccine. I am totally confident there is no link.

Parents who have been frightened by bad press about the MMR vaccine may feel that single vaccines could be safer, but these vaccines are not licensed for use in the UK. They also have to be given some time apart, so you run the risk of leaving your child exposed to these viruses for longer. The MMR can cause swollen glands for a couple of days and a measles-like rash for up to three days, but these are not contagious.

INFLUENZA VACCINE FOR CHILDREN

This vaccine programme is being rolled out. It is given as a nasal spray that contains a live but weakened flu virus, which cannot give children the flu. It may leave children with a runny nose.

HPV VACCINE

The HPV vaccine is given to girls aged 12–13, aiming for them to be vaccinated against the human papilloma virus before they become sexually active and are exposed to the virus. There are over 100 different types of HPV, but the vaccine protects against the two strains responsible for 70% of cervical cancers and against those causing genital warts. It is given as two injections within a 6–24 month period.

MEN. ACWY VACCINE

The Men. ACWY vaccine is given as a single injection into the upper arm. It protects against four bacteria causing meningitis and sepsis (also called septicaemia).

INFLUENZA VACCINE FOR ADULTS

For most of us, flu is a miserable bug that will put us in bed for a couple of weeks but for the elderly and people at risk it can have serious complications; it can even be fatal. Everyone aged over 65, pregnant women, people with long-term health conditions such as asthma, chronic obstructive pulmonary disease (COPD), heart disease, diabetes, kidney disease, liver disease, and certain neurological conditions such as Parkinson's disease and motor neurone disease should all have an annual flu jab. The carers of these patients, and healthcare workers, are also eligible for the vaccination. The flu virus changes each year so a new vaccine is needed annually to protect against the particular strain that is present that year.

SHINGLES VACCINE

The shingles vaccine contains a weakened chickenpox vaccine which means that, very rarely (under 1 in 10,000 people), people may develop a chickenpox-like illness after the vaccine. Having met several elderly patients who have suffered badly from shingles (see below) I would advise anyone who is eligible to accept the vaccine.

DR DAWN'S TOP TIP

We are very lucky here in the UK to have such a comprehensive vaccination schedule, so make the most of it! The NHS doesn't have money to throw around so, if you are offered a vaccination, my advice would be to accept it.

THE ILLNESSES WE VACCINATE AGAINST

DIPHTHERIA

Diphtheria is a highly contagious and potentially fatal condition caused by bacteria that are spread via coughs, sneezes, and by contact with infected people or their clothing. Thanks to the vaccination programme, it is now very rare in the UK.

Symptoms include a high fever (38°C or more), a sore throat with a thick greyish coating at the back of the throat, and problems breathing. It is usually diagnosed with a swab test and needs urgent treatment with antibiotics to prevent potential complications from affecting the heart and nervous system.

TETANUS

Tetanus is caused by bacteria getting into a wound. It is a potentially fatal condition but is now very rare because of the vaccination schedule. I have only ever seen one case of tetanus in my clinical career, and that was when I was working in the Outback in Australia – I looked after an Aboriginal man who developed tetanus after the tribal doctor had packed his leg wound with dried camel dung.

The symptoms of tetanus include a high fever, rapid heartbeat, sweating, and stiffness of the jaw muscles (sometimes referred to as 'lockjaw'). There are often also painful muscle spasms elsewhere in the body. It is treated with tetanus immunoglobulin and antibiotics. Patients often need to be admitted to intensive care.

WHOOPING COUGH (PERTUSSIS)

Whooping cough is another highly contagious disease. It can be diagnosed by the characteristic 'whoop' sound as the individual breathes in after coughing. The early symptoms may seem like any other cough or cold, but as they develop the cough becomes more severe and patients often cough up thick phlegm. Babies under six months old may not make the 'whoop' sound, but you may notice them gagging after coughing bouts, or they may even look as though they have stopped breathing. The cough can last for three months and is treated with antibiotics.

POLIO

Polio has now been eradicated from the UK, thanks to the very successful vaccination programme, and is likely to be eradicated globally in the near future. It is caused by a picornavirus – one of a group of viruses that live in the gut. The virus can be detected in the stools of a polio sufferer up to six weeks after the start of the illness. Around 95% of cases are mild, with no symptoms, or there may be a mild viral illness, but more serious cases affect the brain and spinal cord. In this instance the individual will develop a high fever, headache and stiff neck, and there may be progressive weakness or even paralysis and breathing difficulties if the muscles of the chest wall are involved. It can leave the individual with paralysed limbs that do not develop.

There is no specific treatment for polio, which is why it is so important to be vaccinated.

HAEMOPHILUS INFLUENZA TYPE B INFECTIONS

Haemophilus influenza type B is a bacteria that can cause a number of different problems including meningitis, pneumonia and septicaemia (blood poisoning). It is a very serious infection – 1 in every 20 children who develop Hib meningitis don't survive, and many of those who do survive are left deaf, with learning disabilities or epilepsy. Hib is spread in the same way as coughs and colds but is – thankfully – rare in the UK, since the Hib vaccination has been included in the childhood vaccination programme since 1992.

PNEUMOCOCCAL INFECTIONS

These are caused by a bacteria that can cause a wide variety of infections, the most serious being blood poisoning, pneumonia, meningitis and infections of the bones (osteomyelitis) and joints (septic arthritis)

ROTAVIRUS INFECTIONS

Rotavirus is highly infectious and is easily spread among families. The virus can also survive for several days on surfaces, so personal hygiene and cleaning are crucial if your household is affected. It can cause profuse diarrhoea, which can lead to dehydration.

MENINGITIS

Meningitis is an infection of the membranes that cover the brain (the meninges). It presents with a high fever, but cold hands and feet. Babies may be floppy and listless and off their food. They may give an odd, high-pitched cry and their skin may look blotchy. Meningitis is a medical emergency and needs urgent hospital treatment with antibiotics. About a quarter of children who develop bacterial meningitis will have long-term problems, such as hearing loss, after the infection.

MEASLES

Measles is a highly contagious viral infection. Symptoms usually develop ten days after the initial infection, and start with cold-like symptoms. Sufferers go on to develop sore red eyes and may be sensitive to light. They can have a very high temperature (up to 40°C), and they develop white-greyish spots on the inside of the cheeks, called Koplik's spots. A few days later the classic pink-brown blotchy rash appears. It starts on the head or neck and spreads over the body. Unfortunately, there are some serious complications associated with measles, including meningitis, seizures, hepatitis and blindness. There is also a very rare long-term problem called subacute sclerosing panencephalitis (SSPE) which affects 1 in 25,000 people who have had measles, in which the brain becomes fatally inflamed several years after the initial infection.

MUMPS

Mumps is a viral infection causing swelling of the parotid glands, which are found at the side of the face just in front of the ears. Sufferers may also get a high fever and joint pains. It can also cause swelling of the testicles in boys and the ovaries in girls. An estimated 1 in 10 men experience a drop in their sperm count (the amount of healthy sperm their body can produce) after mumps. However, this is very rarely enough to cause infertility. Very rarely, it can cause a form of meningitis.

RUBELLA

Rubella is another viral infection that can cause a high fever, cold-like symptoms, aching joints, swollen glands and a pink spotty rash. It is spread in the same way as coughs and colds.

If a pregnant woman contracts rubella it can have very serious consequences for the unborn baby, including blindness, deafness, brain damage and heart abnormalities.

SHINGLES

Shingles is caused by the varicella zoster virus, which causes chickenpox. Unlike other viruses, this virus does not clear from the body after infection but climbs back up the nerve endings and becomes dormant. In most people it remains dormant, but about one in four people will have at least one other episode of shingles in their lives. Typically it starts as itchy blisters affecting a strip of skin but not crossing the midline (imagine drawing a vertical line from the top of your head to between your legs, dividing the body in half). The blisters gradually crust over but can be associated with a severe burning pain and tender skin, which can continue for weeks or months after the rash has disappeared. The patient is contagious until the last blister has healed.

TRAVEL VACCINES

The world is undoubtedly becoming a smaller place – but we mustn't allow that to make us complacent about travel health.

Which vaccines you need will depend on where you are going. I flew to Panama last year to Bear Grylls' island to raise money for charity. When I went to have my travel vaccines, I was surprised that I didn't need to take anti-malarial prophylaxis to go to the island I was visiting — but if I had planned to go just a few miles down the coast, I would have needed this. Just because you have been to an area before, don't assume you'll need the same vaccinations. Most surgeries now offer travel health advice with the practice nurse, who has access to the most up-to-date advice on what vaccines you will need, but make sure you leave enough time to have all the vaccines, as some need to be given several weeks apart. Also, make sure you follow the travel clinic's advice to the letter. I met a woman a couple of years ago whose eldest son volunteered at a school in Africa during his gap year. He had a place at university on his return to study sports science, and was a very fit, active young man. When he flew home at the end of the year, he gave his remaining anti-malarial pills to a child at the school who had malaria — because the local doctors couldn't access the medicines the child needed. Sadly, the young man hadn't realised the importance of continuing to take anti-malarial protection for four weeks after returning from a malarial zone. Within a week of his return he was in intensive care with cerebral malaria. Unfortunately, he didn't survive.

DR DAWN'S TOP TIP

Plan ahead if you are travelling. If you are likely to need vaccinations, you will have to include them in your budget. Some vaccines are offered free on the NHS — these include diphtheria, typhoid, hepatitis A and cholera, as these diseases are thought to pose a significant risk to the health of the British public if brought back into the country. But you may be expected to pay for some vaccines, including those to protect against yellow fever, rabies, TB, meningitis, hepatitis B, Japanese encephalitis and tick-borne encephalitis.

CHAPTER 10

MIND OVER MATTER

Clifford Brewer was a distinguished surgeon who had started his training at Liverpool Medical School when he was just fifteen. His lengthy career included spells at the Radcliffe Infirmary in Oxford and at the Royal Liverpool Infirmary, where on one occasion he had to remove an ingrowing toenail from John Lennon's foot. But it was his outstanding record during World War II that earned him a full-page obituary in *The Times*. After the D-Day landings in Normandy, he operated on more than 1,000 battlefield casualties.

When he turned 100 in 2013, he was still enjoying regular visits to Wherwell Lake in Hampshire to pursue his love of fly-fishing. But then he started to decline. 'I'm beginning to feel my years,' he told a BBC reporter soon afterwards. In 2017 he had a party to celebrate his 104th birthday, when he told his grand-daughter Charlotte that he felt it was 'time to go'. He died in his sleep that night.

There is a slightly obscure branch of science called chronopsychology, which looks at the links between the way people think and the timing of things that happen in their lives. It has been shown that people are able to postpone their death until after a major life event or a moment of important emotional significance. For example, three American presidents – John Adams, Thomas Jefferson and James Monroe – all died on the 4th of July, American Independence Day. It's as though they held on to life to ensure they were still there to enjoy the celebrations.

Although it may seem rather sad to die on your birthday, like

Clifford Brewer, it's actually very common. Statistically, you would expect your chance of dying to be the same on every day. But scientists in Switzerland, who studied records of 2.4 million deaths, found that people were actually 18% more likely to die on their birthday than any other day. Some of this may be down to over-zealous birthday celebrations involving excessive indulgence in alcohol, but I believe it has more to do with people having the psychological desire to reach a certain longevity milestone. The birthday itself may be the ideal opportunity to see family and friends one last time. As psychologist Professor Richard Wiseman puts it: 'You are knife-edged on death, and you kept yourself going until your birthday. You think, "That's it, I've had enough, I'm out of here".'[1]

Either way, if you die on your birthday you're in good company – William Shakespeare, Ingrid Bergman, Arnold Bennett and F.D. Roosevelt are some of the better known people who died on the same date as they were born.

DON'T WORRY, BE HAPPY

So far I have written about the links between various physical conditions and human longevity. In this chapter I'm going to show that psychological factors also have a major part to play in determining a person's well-being and how likely they are to live to a good age. Your outlook on life, how optimistic you are, and the quality and frequency of your relationships with other people are all major factors.

It will come as no surprise that happiness is good for your health. There have been numerous studies to support this, including a recent one conducted at University College London.[2] The UCL team followed the progress of 3,800 people aged 52 to 79 and asked them to rate their level of happiness on a scale from 1 to 5. To get a more accurate measure, they asked the participants to assess their happiness rating on several occasions, at different times of day, and over an extended period of time. Five years later, just 3.6% of the participants in the top happiness group had died. In contrast, some 7.3% of the people in the lowest group had died. After accounting for all other factors, including depression and state of physical health, the researchers concluded that the happiest people were more than a third less likely to die.

Our level of happiness seems to have a direct effect on how well our bodies function. For example, it's been shown that happier people have a lower heart rate – about six beats per minute slower – than unhappy people. Tests also show that increased happiness leads to lower blood pressure, a more robust immune system and a much lower chance of suffering from chronic pain. Happy people are also more likely to take better care of themselves, exercise regularly, avoid unhealthy foods and get regular medical check-ups.

So if happiness can make such a difference to people's well-being, shouldn't we be more aware of it as a public health issue? In one country, it already is. Bhutan is a small Buddhist kingdom set high in the Himalayan mountains between India and China. In 2008 the country's government rejected Gross Domestic Product (GDP) as the best way of tracking economic progress. Instead it amended the country's constitution to introduce the GNH, a measure of their citizens' Gross National Happiness. The government believes that well-being is more important than material growth. In Bhutan's schools, children take part in daily meditation classes and periods of listening to soothing traditional music. A GNH Commission oversees all Bhutan's government decisions, either approving or rejecting them, depending on whether or not they will improve happiness levels. To assess how well it is doing, the government regularly conducts surveys of its people, asking them detailed questions about their economic well-being, their local community, their interactions with friends and neighbours, their participation in cultural events and their state of mind.

Bhutan's initiative was originally considered to be slightly eccentric, but the idea that national happiness is important and measurable has started to spread. Since 2012 a committee linked to the United Nations has published an annual World Happiness Report (http://worldhappiness.report/). Table 10.1 shows the countries with the world's highest happiness scores, according to the committee's most recent report.

Table 10.1: The happiest countries in the world. Reproduced from Helliwell, J., Layard, R. & Sachs, J. (2017). World Happiness Report 2017, New York: Sustainable Development Solutions Network.

Overall rank	Change in rank	Country
1	▲ 3	Norway
2	▼ -1	Denmark
3	– 0	Iceland
4	▼ -2	Switzerland
5	– 0	Finland
6	▲ 1	Netherlands
7	▼ -1	Canada
8	– 0	New Zealand
9	– 0	Australia
10	– 0	Sweden

The ranking is based on detailed analysis of a range of factors, including GDP per person, life expectancy, people's freedom to make life choices, levels of corruption, and subjective assessments of factors like trust and generosity. The UK comes in at number 19. The Central African Republic comes last, at number 155.

The idea that having a positive outlook on life can have direct medical benefits was recently tested by the British Heart Foundation. It assessed the mental attitudes of a group of 396 patients who had been admitted to hospital following a heart attack or serious angina attack. They found that the most pessimistic patients were twice as likely to die or need further surgery over the next four years than the most optimistic. This is partly because the optimists were much more likely to heed good advice, such as to eat more fruit and vegetables.

The British Heart Foundation's associate medical director, Dr Mike Knapton, said: 'The next steps for this research would be to show that psychotherapy to improve optimism can improve the outcomes for pessimistic people. Suffering from a serious condition such as a heart attack or angina can take a drastic emotional toll, which we know can lead to depression, further lowering the chances of a full recovery.'[3]

DR DAWN'S TOP TIP

You could say that whether you're an optimist or a pessimist is down to the character you inherited at birth, and there's nothing you can do to change your outlook on life. But there's one easy way to lift your mood: take regular exercise. Studies have shown that physical activity is a more powerful and effective treatment for overcoming negativity and boosting self-esteem than any other relaxation technique. Yet another reason to get fit!

IN SICKNESS AND IN HEALTH

There are a number of factors that affect individual happiness and therefore also longevity. Some of these we can control, while others are much harder to change even if we wanted to. Marriage is a good place to start.

In 1858 a British scientist called William Farr set out to investigate the 'conjugal condition' of the adult population. He divided his research subjects into three groups: 'married', 'celibate' or 'widowed'. Using birth, death and marriage records, he discovered that those who were unmarried died 'in undue proportion' to their married counterparts. Farr's was the first scholarly work to suggest that married people live longer, healthier lives.

'Marriage is a healthy estate,' he concluded. 'The single individual is more likely to be wrecked on his voyage than the lives joined together in matrimony.'[4] Well, that's one way of putting it.

Since then dozens more research projects all over the world have provided proof of the 'marriage advantage' – the fact that married people live longer than their unmarried peers. It's been shown that in the UK married couples tend to smoke and drink less than unmarried people. Being in a happy marriage means you have a partner to provide emotional support and companionship – and married people can benefit from 'positive nagging', where one partner encourages the other to eat properly, keep physically fit, or visit the doctor when necessary.

Marriage seems to have a directly beneficial effect on physical health, with married people having reduced instances of cancer, high blood pressure, pneumonia, Alzheimer's, type 2 diabetes and depression. Married people are 71% more likely to survive a stroke, and 14% more likely to survive a heart attack, than unmarried people.

Interestingly, it is men who benefit most from being married. Figures from the Office of National Statistics showed that the mortality rate for married men aged between 30 and 59 was less than half that for those who were unmarried. For women, there was hardly any difference at all.

In the UK, around four in every ten marriages end in divorce. If your marriage ends you are statistically at greater risk than your single peers. Research by the American Center for the Study of Aging[5] found that the death rate for men who had divorced in the previous nine years was 37% higher than for a similarly aged group who remained married. Divorce is also linked to a higher rate of suicide in men – though not in women. But all is not lost: according to the American study, if divorced men over 50 remarry or find a new long-term partner, their health level goes right back up to where it would have been if they'd stayed married.

In health terms, there is one downside to marriage. Married people are about 25% more likely to be obese or overweight compared to their unmarried peers. This may be because once people have found a long-term partner, they 'let themselves go' as they are no longer on the market, trying to attract a mate. But, on balance, being married or in a happy long-term relationship is definitely good for your health.

THE SCIENCE OF SEX

Whether you're single or attached, there's one thing you can do to boost your longevity: have sex. There are several reasons why sexual activity can have a directly beneficial effect on your well-being:

Immunity. People who have sex a couple of times a week have higher amounts of the antibody immunoglobulin A (IgA) than those who have sex less than once a week. igA is one of the body's natural defences against colds and flu.

Fitness. Sex is a form of exercise, so it increases your blood flow and gets your heart pumping, although it doesn't actually help you burn off that many calories (see Chapter 6).

Heart. Regular sexual activity reduces the risk of cardiovascular disease and strokes.

Dementia. According to American research, having regular sex helps us grow new brain cells. It seems that, the more sex you have, the more cells you can grow. So sex can protect your brain against decline.

Pain. During sex the hormone oxytocin (sometimes called the 'cuddle hormone') is released in your body. This can reduce physical pain, including headaches.

Sleep. Oxytocin also promotes better sleep. For men a powerful
   orgasm is the equivalent of taking a 2 mg shot of diazepam.
   That's why men often fall asleep soon after sex.
Prostate cancer. An Australian study[6] found that men aged 20 to
   50 who ejaculate at least five times a week were much less
   likely to get prostate cancer when they got older.
Mood. A healthy sex life tends to boost self-confidence, as well as
   making people feel happier and more contented.

There is also evidence that having regular sex improves cognition,
promotes bone growth, maintains and repairs tissues, and keeps your
skin looking healthy and supple. However, I should strike a note of
caution: this may be a case where cause and effect are the wrong
way round. You could argue that people who are healthier to begin
with are more likely to have an active sex life than those who are
weak or unhealthy. Either way, sex is good for you and it could
prolong your life.

WITH A LITTLE HELP FROM YOUR FRIENDS

If being married or in a long-term relationship can be good for
your health, so too can having children. A Swedish study of 1.4
million adults published in 2017[7] found that at 60 years of age the
life expectancy of men who had children was two years greater
than that of their childless counterparts. For women the gap was
1.5 years. The study also found that the longevity benefit becomes
greater as you get older. Interestingly, widows and widowers also
live longer if they have a family. This suggests that children become
even more important for staying alive if your spouse is no longer
around.

When you first have children, the advantages may be unclear –

who needs sleep deprivation, constant caregiving, a reduced disposable income, and having to put up with intermittent or constant whinging? But although parenting may on occasions drive you crazy, if you get through those difficult first years, there are long-term benefits!

So families, sexual relationships and children are all beneficial. However, having a good network of friends and neighbours can be equally effective. This is the conclusion of a huge study of over 300,000 people worldwide conducted by a team from Brigham Young University in Utah, USA.[8] They calculated that having few friends is as damaging to your health as smoking 15 cigarettes a day or being an alcoholic. As the lead researcher Julianne Holt-Lunstad put it: 'When someone is connected to a group and feels responsibility for other people, that sense of purpose and meaning translates to taking better care of themselves and taking fewer risks.' In mortality terms, people with the strongest social networks were nearly twice as likely to be alive at any given age as those who were lonely. This finding applied to people of all ages and backgrounds, irrespective of their initial health status. The larger and more varied your social network, the happier and the healthier you are likely to be.

The nature of friendship tends to change with time. Many people in their twenties and thirties can boast of having 1,000+ 'friends' on Facebook (the average for all Facebook users is 130). As we get older we tend to have fewer, but closer, friends. A British biologist, Robin Dunbar, thinks people can have a maximum of around 150 friends, defining them as 'those people with whom you have a personalised relationship, one that is reciprocal and based around general obligations of trust and reciprocity'. Most people have an inner circle of around five 'close friends' then, as the number gets larger, the level of contact and emotional intimacy decreases. But whether they really are friends or just acquaintances, throughout our lives these social relationships are vital to our physical and mental well-being.[9]

Conversely, loneliness is strongly linked to depression, anxiety and ill health. According to Age UK, one in ten people over 65 say they often or always feel lonely. The problem tends to be more common in men than women, and it particularly affects people who have, or had, low incomes. Many people struggle to maintain social networks because friends and partners die, they stop working, or they have mobility problems. Also, people who move away from home to go abroad or live by the sea often live to regret it (see Chapter 11). One recent study concluded that loneliness is twice as deadly as obesity.[10]

DR DAWN'S TOP TIP

Most people aren't lonely when they are young or in middle age, so it's worth trying to plan ways in which you could stay socially active as you get older. For example, people who are married should not always rely on their partner to make all their social arrangements; if that person dies or you divorce, you could find your social network has disappeared. You're never too old to take up new hobbies, join new interest groups, learn a new skill, or get involved with a local charity. And don't be afraid to embrace technology; 102-year-old Jimmy Thirsk (who we met in Chapter 1) told me that he uses the internet every day to keep in touch with family members and former work colleagues all over the world.

Of course, if you want to live a long and healthy life, you could simply pray that this will happen. A number of studies have been carried out on religious service attendance and longevity. According to a recent paper published by Harvard University,[11] people who regularly attend a place of worship (of whatever kind) are less likely to get depression, have a much lower risk of suicide, and generally have reduced mortality rates at any particular age.

Some religious people would suggest that this is because they have been blessed with the gift of a longer and healthier life by some higher power. But the explanation is probably more mundane.

By attending religious services you are participating in a group activity that enhances your social connections and sense of belonging to a community. Also many religions encourage their followers to practise a healthy lifestyle – so abstinence from alcohol, periods of fasting and various types of meditation can clearly be beneficial from a medical point of view.

PAWS FOR THOUGHT

If your social network is not as extensive as it should be, a quick and effective solution is available: get a pet. The health benefits of owning an animal have been proven beyond doubt. Pet owners tend to visit their doctors less often than people without pets, and are less likely to suffer from depression. Stroking a pet reduces levels of the stress hormone cortisol, and can also lower heart rates and blood pressure levels.

If you own a dog it probably expects to 'go walkies' on a regular basis, so that encourages you to exercise, and meeting other dog walkers enhances your social circle. Animals are calming, accepting friends that usually offer unconditional love and kindness – and if they can also improve your health and well-being, then so much the better.

The Royal College of Nursing is so convinced about the benefits of 'animal therapy' that it has begun to encourage hospitals to allow pets to visit their owners while they are convalescing. They say there is clear evidence that patients who have visits from their pets tend to be more physically active, have reduced anxiety and to recover more quickly. Of course, there are concerns that bringing animals into hospitals can spread infections, but there is considerable evidence from other countries that the benefits can outweigh the risks. Bringing pets into children's hospitals has been found to be particularly effective in raising the spirits of younger patients.

HARD LABOUR

People often complain that their job is killing them. Unfortunately, if you suffer from work-related stress, this could be true. Stress leads your adrenal glands to release glucocorticoid hormones, which are thought to damage the body's DNA. It can also produce a range of emotional symptoms, including loss of motivation or confidence, as well as an inability to concentrate or make decisions. Someone who is over-stressed may also become more visibly anxious or nervous, change their eating habits, get regular headaches, or start taking lots of time off work. In severe cases, stress can lead to depression or suicide. People feel stressed when their work demands exceed their ability to cope.

Worse still, work-related stress can affect groups of people as well as individuals. Poor morale, bad management or unpleasant working conditions can cause entire companies to be blighted by employee stress. I certainly know lots of people who have had the misfortune to work in places like this. An unhappy workplace is much more likely to be an unhealthy workplace too. In the UK about 12 million working days are lost each year to work-related stress. That makes it the biggest single reason why people take sick leave, beating all other medical conditions, and accounting for an estimated £57 billion a year in lost productivity. No line of work seems to be immune to the problem, my own profession being a prime example. In 2017 the British Medical Association reported that over half of our GPs and locums had been unwell during the previous year because of stress. One in ten had taken time off as a result.

Work-related stress could also be one of the main reasons that the life expectancy gap between the sexes is closing. In the UK, men still live about 3.7 years less than women (see Chapter 1), but their life expectancy is catching up. One reason for this is that men are healthier because of the decline in punishing jobs, such as coal mining or working in heavy industry. Meanwhile there has been a trend for women to move from non-working roles into challenging careers, with even more stress for those who combine work with raising a family.

DR DAWN'S TOP TIP

If you think your health is suffering because of work-related stress, you need to change the way you work or the environment you work in. Although each workplace is different, here are some general rules:

- Learn to say 'no' if you can't take on extra work or responsibility. You need to become empowered to set your own limits, even if it risks antagonising your employer.

- If possible, reduce your workload. Many people are perfectionists who find it very hard to delegate tasks to others. Sometime you need to learn to let go.

- Try to make your working environment as comfortable as possible. Improved lighting, ventilation or more comfortable seating could help.

- If possible, work regular hours, and make sure you take the breaks and holidays you're entitled to.

- Take a walk or get some fresh air during the working day. Lunch doesn't have to take an hour – simply taking a break is important.

- Learn to speak out and share your problems with others. Discussing issues with colleagues can be helpful.

- If all else fails, leave and work elsewhere. A job that damages your physical or mental health is ultimately not worth having.

Legally, employers must look after their staff. A failure to do so can result in claims from employees for personal injury, discrimination or constructive dismissal. In extreme cases the employer could face a criminal prosecution from the Health and Safety Executive. However, any sensible employer should realise that a happier and healthier workplace is also a more productive workplace – so everyone wins.

Your choice of profession can be a major factor in predicting your health and lifespan. Even when you've retired, the job you did in the past will still affect the length of your future. According to the Office of National Statistics, professionals such as lawyers or accountants will typically outlive builders and cleaners by an average of eight years. This is not just because office jobs generally put less strain on people, but also because they offer people more autonomy and control over what they do.

Not all stress is necessarily bad. In recent years, there has been a lot of discussion about 'good stress' versus 'bad stress'. Bad stress is characterised by a feeling that you have no control, and it can last for days or even years. On the other hand, good stress occurs when you have to face problems that you *can* solve, and it doesn't usually last very long. Psychologist Dr Kelly McGonigal puts it like this: 'We are born with so many instincts for thriving under stress. If you can view stress differently, as it's happening, you can alter the effect it has on you. The key is changing how we think about it. If you embrace stress, you can transform fear into courage, isolation into connection, and suffering into meaning.'[12]

One American study[13] that tracked 30,000 people found that people who reported experiencing a damaging level of stress in their lives had a 43% higher mortality rate in the following eight years than the average population. Meanwhile, those who said they were under stress but that they were perfectly able to cope were actually less likely to die than average – including those who said that their lives were relatively stress-free. So the old saying that 'what doesn't kill you makes you stronger' may well be true.

DR DAWN'S TOP TIP

Your instinct may be to see any stress as something negative. But if you change your thinking to see any stress as a positive, you can regain control and take the necessary steps to overcome that challenge and bounce back quickly. Anxiety and excitement are two sides of the same coin, and dealing with a series of short-term stresses make us more focused, productive and resilient.

If work can be bad for you, so too can giving up work. The writer Saul Bellow was suitably scathing about the idea. 'Retirement is an illusion,' he said. 'Not a reward but a mantrap. The bankrupt underside of success. A shortcut to death. Golf courses are too much like cemeteries.'[14]

For many people the idea of retirement means the welcome prospect of enjoying 'golden years' of endless leisure. For others, giving up work represents a loss of self-esteem, resulting in poorer physical or mental health. We often read about people who have retired and then died shortly afterwards because they felt they had nothing left to live for.

But it's really a matter of choice. If you love your job, why would you want to stop? I can't imagine David Attenborough announcing that he is retiring from making nature documentaries. Similarly, if you have spent many decades working in a menial or unsatisfying role, why would you continue any longer than you have to? In longevity terms, there's no evidence to suggest that one path is intrinsically better than the other. An American study[15] found that people who worked longer had an 11% lower mortality risk than those who took early retirement. However, an Israeli study[16] found that people who retired early had the same lifespan as those who did not – and a German study[17] concluded that people who retire before the age of 61 live longer than those who continue to work. So this is clearly a case of 'you pays your money and you takes your choice!'

DR DAWN'S TOP TIP

If you suffer from stress – because of your job or for any other reason – you should consider taking up some form of meditation.

Medical science has long understood that people who meditate regularly tend to be healthier and have a more positive outlook on life. It seems that meditation encourages the body to produce more of an enzyme called telomerase, which helps repair the telomeres on your chromosomes (see Chapter 2). The benefits seem to apply to all popular types of meditation, including mindfulness, transcendental meditation, qigong, zazen or Kundalini. You can find out more about these types of meditation (and several others) online.

A WORKOUT AT THE MIND GYM

Chapter 1 looked at how your biological age can differ from your actual age. In the same way, doctors can analyse your brain to find out whether it is 'older' or 'younger' than you are. A team of neuroscientists from Imperial College London[18] used MRI scans to predict people's ages, based on their volume of brain tissue. They found that those whose brains appeared older than their true age were more likely to die early, as well as being in worse physical and mental health.

In a separate study, researchers at University College London[19] discovered that London's black cab drivers have a larger posterior hippocampus than non-cab drivers. This part of the brain is associated with long-term memory. To become a London cabbie you have to master 'the knowledge' – a detailed understanding of the thousands of roads and routes throughout London. The researchers also found that the longer the cab drivers had been doing the job, the larger their posterior hippocampus grew. This suggests that the brain is like a muscle – the more you exercise it, the bigger it gets.

There is some evidence that your brain can benefit from mental exercise in the same way that your body benefits from physical exercise. If your brain gets a workout, it can grow new neural connections and strengthen weak ones. But the key is to make your brain do something new, and maybe something difficult. Repeating something you already know will have little effect. The more you use your brain, the more you'll protect it against the risk of memory loss. Keeping your mind fit and active also reduces the risk that you will get dementia. As the old saying goes, 'if you don't use it, you'll lose it'.

DR DAWN'S TOP TIP

Not surprisingly, a whole industry has sprung up based on the idea that you can attend a 'gym for the mind'. There are online courses, brain-training counsellors and a variety of apps that make wild promises about the transformative effect they will have on your life. But you don't need to spend a small fortune on brain-training gurus. There are lots of simple ways to keep your mind alert:

- Set yourself mental challenges; for example try counting backwards from 100 in 2s, 3s or 4s. Gradually make these challenges more difficult.
- Try mental puzzles such as jigsaws, Sudoku, chess, bridge or crosswords.
- Memorise things. Learning a poem or a song off by heart is an excellent way to exercise your mind muscles, and it could be the basis of an entertaining party piece.
- Wean yourself off using a calculator. When checking receipts or restaurant bills, try doing the adding up in your head.
- It's never too late to learn a language – and it's most useful if you learn a language that's spoken in a country you're likely to visit. (Bilingual people have been found to have a lower risk of developing Alzheimer's disease.)

- Take up a new creative hobby, such as painting, photography or playing a musical instrument. The brains of professional musicians have been found to have a larger volume of grey matter than those of non-musicians.[20]

Chapter 11 discusses a place where people live longer than they do anywhere else in Europe. As you will see, happiness, strong personal relationships, and a lack of stress play a very important part in this longevity.

CHAPTER 11
A PLACE TO
GROW OLD

It's a sunny spring morning, and I'm travelling along a narrow, winding road that skirts the Italian coast to the south of Salerno. The countryside is typical of the region: medieval towns cling to rocky hillsides on my left, while far below me on my right the sea appears intermittently as a rippling jewel-blue blanket. Everything here looks wonderful – not least because of the bright Mediterranean sunshine that bathes the scene. Not surprisingly, this has been designated an Area of Outstanding Natural Beauty.

My destination is a small port called Acciaroli. According to local legend, author Ernest Hemingway came to stay here in 1951. He apparently based the 'old man' in his Pulitzer Prize-winning novel, *The Old Man and the Sea*, on a resident of Acciaroli. But over the past few years Acciaroli has become famous worldwide for a very different reason – the longevity of its people.

Acciaroli and the surrounding villages belong to the municipality of Pollica. The total population numbers around 2,000. Of these, 10% – some 200 people – are over 100 years old. Consider just how remarkable this is: it's about 500 times higher than the average for the UK. Or, to put it another way, imagine arriving in London to find that its population includes one million centenarians! The pattern of ageing in Acciaroli is also unusual because its men are living just as long as its women: of the people aged over 90, there is roughly an equal number of males and females.

Not surprisingly, Acciaroli has become the subject of major

scientific interest. In 2016 a team of researchers from San Diego School of Medicine and the Sapienza University in Rome arrived to conduct a detailed study of the local citizens. They spent six months in the area, taking blood samples from around 80 people and assessing all the factors that could be causing this statistical phenomenon.

It's also significant that the people here are not just living very long lives, but most of them are in excellent health. There's no such thing as an old people's home in Acciaroli, and the nearest hospital is 40 miles away.

I wanted to find out more about Acciaroli's remarkable citizens for myself. So, accompanied by my wonderful interpreter, Emilio, I went to meet some of them. The people I met were happy to tell me about their long lives.

Giuseppe Vassallo meets me at a café in the centre of the village. He uses a walking stick, but that's not really unusual for someone approaching his century. Giuseppe tells me that in his family there's nothing remarkable about longevity: 'My brother lived to 103, my cousin is 101. All my seven brothers and sisters have lived to over 90.' But he says that most of his life has been very tough: 'When I was young we were really poor and life was very sad. There was no light, no electricity. My friend and I had to walk every day to the next village to go to school, without shoes. When I tell my children about these things, they simply don't believe me. If you ask me what job I used to do, I tell you I have done everything in my time – I did whatever it took to earn some money just to get by.'

Giuseppe left Acciaroli when his wife died eight years ago. But then he decided to move back, and he thinks it's the best decision he ever made. 'We are in a place where there is sea air and it keeps everything clean and fresh. For example, I've noticed that when [my nephew] comes to visit me from his home in the north of Italy, he looks sad and run down. But after just one week here he looks completely different – more alive. It's the good quality of the air, I'm sure of it.'

He also attributes his good health to growing his own vegetables and eating a diet that's high in olive oil. And since he returned to Acciaroli he has also found a new companion: 'I found a young girl. Well, when I say she's a young girl, she's 50 years old. But I like spending time with her and that's made things much better. I've found that being in love really helps. It makes me feel like I'm born again. In my own mind I'm still young; I don't feel old at all.'

Just a few yards from the café, in a narrow street behind the harbour, I visit one of Acciaroli's oldest married couples. Amina Fedullo is 95 and her husband Antonio is 101. They were married in 1950. They sit together in their small kitchen, where they have just enjoyed a home-cooked lunch. 'I cook all the time,' Amina tells me. 'Every day he looks at the clock and says "It's twelve o'clock – where's my pasta?" Then later on, at about five or six o'clock, he says it again: "Where's my dinner?" Maybe it's having to put up with him nagging me every day that's kept me alive for so long!'

Antonio agrees that some friendly confrontation is helpful for maintaining a long and successful marriage. 'Life isn't any fun if you don't have arguments. But when we fight it doesn't last very long.'

Just like Giuseppe, Antonio and Amina tell me that their early life was pretty tough. Antonio was called up to serve in the Italian army when Mussolini was in power. He was sent to fight in the Second Italo-Abyssinian War (1935–6): 'The temperature was never below 40 degrees, and I saw a lot of terrible things.' But eventually he came back to his birthplace, Acciaroli, and started work as a fisherman. That's when he met Amina, who recalls the moment in a poem she recites to me from memory:

By the sea, the waves put my soul at rest.
I saw a little boat approach, a fisherman laying nets.
When he got closer, I looked at him and he smiled at me.
He invited me on board for a ride. It was a pleasure trip.
I was taken by the beauty of the sea, and I became the
    bride of the fisherman.[1]

So do they have any theories about the Acciaroli phenomenon? Amina believes the air quality plays a large part: 'The air is pure because it's fresh air from the sea. Even inland you can feel it, and the grass has a different smell.' Antonio has a different view: 'Our diet must be an important factor. We eat much more fish than red meat. We've always made our own olive oil. Everything we eat is clean and natural; we eat fresh fruit directly from the trees.'

So is that the secret? Is eating the right food one of the main reasons they're living such long and healthy lives?

THE MEDITERRANEAN DIET

Most people have heard of the Mediterranean diet, and you probably have some idea of what it entails – eating lots of fresh fruit and vegetables, eating fish rather than meat, consuming healthy salads soaked in olive oil, and avoiding sugary foods such as cakes and biscuits. What I didn't know before I visited Acciaroli is that the diet has its origins right here in this region of Italy. And the story of the man who first described the diet has particular relevance to the subject of longevity.

Just a couple of miles down the coast from Acciaroli, in the seaside village of Pioppi, is a splendid museum that's housed in a seventeenth-century palace. It's the Museum of the Mediterranean Diet. On the day I went, large groups of schoolchildren were busy learning about different types of foods and drawing pictures of healthy ingredients. There are displays showing herbs and spices, and the range of nuts you can find growing locally, as well as information about the economic, historical and geographic aspects of the area.

Much of the museum is dedicated to Ancel Keys, who described the diet. Born in Colorado Springs, USA, in 1904, Keys was an interesting character. He originally studied political science and economics at the University of California before deciding to turn his attention to biology, oceanography and human physiology. He took particular interest in dietary and nutritional science, and during World War II he helped the US government work out 'K-rations' – the meals American soldiers took on active service. These meals were hailed as a great success and became a major part of military nutrition in subsequent years.

Keys had heard that people in this part of Italy had a record of living long and healthy lives, so in 1962 he moved to Pioppi to research the factors that contributed to their health and longevity. He described the local community as his 'living laboratory'. Eventually he documented his findings in his 1975 book *How to Eat Well and Stay Well the Mediterranean Way*, co-written with his wife Margaret, who was also an expert on biochemistry and nutrition. Their main conclusion was that saturated fats of the type found in milk and meat have adverse effects, particularly on the body's cardiovascular system. Meanwhile, unsaturated fats of the type found in vegetable oils were beneficial. Before the book was published, there was a widespread belief that all fat was unhealthy, whereas Key showed that there were 'good fats' and 'bad fats', a view that is still commonly held today.

The museum shows how the Mediterranean diet can be represented by a pyramid (Figure 11.1). At the bottom of the pyramid are large quantities of fresh fruit and vegetables, as well as bread, olive oil, seeds, herbs and spices. Further up – and in smaller quantities – are fish and seafood. Above this are poultry, eggs, cheese and yoghurt. Right at the top in the smallest triangle are 'meats and sweets'. The idea is that although it's OK to eat everything, the ratio in which you consume different foods should reflect their position on the pyramid: eat lots of fruit and vegetables, while saving the less healthy meats and sweets for special occasions. Ancel Keys also said that alcohol could be beneficial, particularly if consumed as a moderate quantity of red wine. His book contained a large number of recipes for healthy Mediterranean meals, all of which Ancel and Margaret Keys had tested in their own Italian kitchen.

Figure 11.1: The food pyramid of the Mediterranean diet.

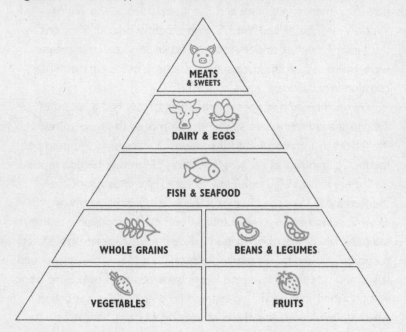

Ancel Keys practised what he preached. After the book became a worldwide bestseller, he boasted that he would live 20 years longer than the average lifespan. To this end he carried on living in Italy and stuck to the principles of the Mediterranean diet. Although he did eventually move back to America, he did achieve his ambition: he died in 2004 just two weeks before his 101st birthday.

This is perhaps the best evidence for why Acciaroli's citizens live such long and healthy lives. Surely it cannot just be a coincidence that the very place with the greatest longevity anywhere in Europe is also where a very successful and popular diet was first identified? It seems to me that the Mediterranean diet has a lot going for it.

ROSEMARY AND TIME

The ongoing research project into Acciaroli's ageing population is being led by Dr Alan Maisel of the San Diego School of Medicine. He decided to investigate the longevity phenomenon after he first visited the area in 2016 and saw no obvious clues as to what was causing it. 'What shocked me is that I don't see people jogging,' he said. 'I do not see people in active exercise classes. I don't see them swimming laps in the ocean.'[2]

As I walk around the village I am also struck by the fact that a lot of Acciaroli's elderly residents are overweight. Many are smoking and drinking, and what they're drinking isn't just red wine.

But Dr Maisel has found that the local population is indeed measurably healthier than the average. There is very little heart disease, and hardly anyone has Alzheimer's. 'We notice that they don't suffer from cataracts,' he said. 'Most people in the US, if you are over 80, have cataracts. We saw none. The goal of this long-term study is to find out why [these people] are living so long by conducting a full genetic analysis and examining lifestyle behaviours.'[3]

The community is also notable for its high level of social interaction. I see groups of elderly residents sitting outside in the spring sun, playing cards. Children tend to stay living near their parents so they are on hand to care for them in their old age. According to Dr Maisel, that's not all: 'Sexual activity among the elderly appears to be rampant. Maybe living long has something to do with that. It's probably the good air and the joie de vivre.'[4]

It may be some years before the results of Dr Maisel's Acciaroli research project are known, and of course there's always the possibility that the reason for Acciaroli's success remains a mystery. However, one early finding from the study has already attracted a lot of attention: it seems the local diet uses a lot of one particular herb – rosemary. Because it's freely available and tastes delicious, locals use liberal quantities of rosemary in their cooking, whether it's to enhance the taste of grilled fish, pasta or a traditional stew.

Acciaroli's mayor, Stefano Pisani, shows me the harbour where large flowerbeds full of rosemary grow on every side. 'Local people really believe in the power of this herb,' he tells me. 'It's like a shield that protects you from all sorts of diseases.'

Rosemary is a good source of calcium, iron and vitamin B6. We also know that it contains carnosic acid, which has been shown to improve mental health and vision. Other research suggests that rosemary has antioxidant, anti-inflammatory and tumour-fighting properties. The rosemary that grows in Acciaroli also benefits from the sunshine and the climate – in warm places such Mediterranean herbs tend to produce higher concentrations of volatile oils, making them much stronger and more flavoursome than the varieties you find in the UK.

Whether eating rosemary eventually turns out to be significant in the quest for a long and healthy life remains to be seen – but adding some rosemary to meals you cook at home won't do any harm.

DR DAWN'S TOP TIP

You could do what Ancel Keys did and move to Acciaroli. Failing that, you could follow the example of its citizens in your quest for a long and healthy life:

- Follow the Mediterranean diet.
- Live near the sea to benefit from the fresh, clean air.
- Keep your children living nearby.
- Maintain an active social life in the local community.
- Stay active, walking and gardening.
- Drink red wine in moderation.
- Enjoy a healthy and active sex life.
- Eat lots of rosemary!

LONGEVITY HOT SPOTS

Acciaroli is Europe's best-known longevity hotspot, but around the world there are several others. Perhaps the most surprising is Loma Linda, a relatively small city in San Bernardino County, the USA, a large area with around two million inhabitants who do not generally live longer than average. Although in Spanish Loma Linda means 'lovely hill', it looks like many other American cities, with a proliferation of convenience stores and fast-food restaurants. But Loma Linda's inhabitants live around ten years longer than most Americans – and, like in Acciaroli, they enjoy better health in their later years.

However, the community in Loma Linda is far from typical. Around half of its 24,000 inhabitants are Seventh-day Adventists, followers of a type of evangelical Christianity that has strict rules about food, exercise and rest. As early as 1864, one of the church's founders, Ellen White, described tobacco as a 'slow, insidious malignant poison'. That's over 80 years before the full dangers of smoking were properly recognised by medical science. The perceptive Mrs White also warned people that alcohol damaged the brain and that eating too much salt is bad for you.

Today the Adventists' lifestyle involves a mostly plant-based diet, regular exercise and a commitment to observe every Sunday as a day of rest. Dr Larry Beeson, a professor at Loma Linda University, has been studying his local community for over 50 years.[5] He believes the vegetarian diet is the main cause of their health and well-being. 'When we look at just mortality, Adventists appear to die of the same diseases, but the age at which they die is much later,' he says. 'The more flesh foods you eat, the more Alzheimer's, the more heart disease, the more cancer, the earlier death occurs. So as people move more towards meat consumption, there tends to be more adverse health outcomes. Whereas going in the other direction, and removing flesh foods from your diet, tends to lead to a delay in the onset of these diseases.'[6]

One 101-year-old inhabitant, Betty Streifling, put her longevity down to 'living a pure life – no alcohol, no tobacco, going to bed early, praising God for his goodness and for the blessing of life'. The Loma Linda lifestyle may not be to everyone's taste, but it does seem to add up to a powerful recipe for well-being.

If you don't fancy living in Acciaroli or Loma Linda, here are a few other places where life expectancies are significantly longer than the average:

Bama – A semi-tropical region in south-west China that is cut off by the mountains. Here, longevity could be linked to the fact that inhabitants get plenty of aerobic exercise. Children climb the mountain to get to school, while adults climb up and down to tend to their crops.

Hunza – This valley in north-east Pakistan is said to be the inspiration for the original Shangri-La. Researchers who visited Hunza found that cancer rates were zero, and that digestive disorders such as ulcers, appendicitis and colitis also did not exist.

Okinawa – A chain of exotic coral-fringed islands in Japan. A study of 600 Okinawa centenarians[7] found that their longevity could be attributed to eating a mainly plant-based diet, supplemented with fish. They also have close social networks, and many of them take the opportunity to exercise outside in the readily available sunshine and fresh air.

Nicoya – This is an 80-mile-long peninsula in Costa Rica, just south of the Nicaraguan border. Nicoya's water has a very high calcium content, which helps promote stronger bones and could reduce the rate of heart disease. It is also a close community, where the elderly people tend to live with their children or grandchildren.

However, you don't necessarily have to emigrate to boost your chances of living a longer life. The place with the highest life expectancy in the UK is Montacute, a village in Somerset with a population of about 700. Here life expectancy is around 89 years – eight years above the UK national average. Many Montacute villagers believe their health and longevity is because they grow their own fruit and vegetables.

The research that identified Montacute as 'Britain's Acciaroli' was carried out by Matthew Edwards, a business consultant. 'These findings show vividly that postcodes can explain substantial variations in mortality,' he said. 'These variations in life expectancy are due to substantial differences in general health and lifestyle patterns between different parts of the UK. The north–south divide in particular is very striking.'[8]

Glasgow currently has the lowest life expectancy in the UK at around 73 years, some 16 years less than the people of Montacute can expect.

SOMETHING IN THE AIR

One of the major factors that significantly affects the health and wellbeing of the local community in different parts of the UK is the level of air pollution. According to John Middleton, President of the Faculty of Public Health, 'It affects everybody. It's affecting children and unborn children, and people who don't have a say in where they live or whether their streets are polluted. It's a universal threat that isn't determined by your personal choice of what you drink or smoke or eat.'[9]

His research suggests that in the UK this pollution is directly responsible for 40,000 deaths every year. 'If you put something in the water that killed 40,000 people a year there would be an outcry,' he says. 'But we put it in the air and we're not doing anything about it. This is a major issue.'

Scientists believe that the risk caused by pollution is similar to that of passive smoking. For example, living next to a dual carriageway is equivalent to being exposed to second-hand smoke from ten cigarettes a day. Now that cigarettes have been banned from workplaces and indoor public spaces, there is a growing demand for stricter laws to improve the quality of our air, particularly in large cities.

In December 1952 a thick, grimy smog descended on London. A blanket of soot hung over the streets, reducing visibility to just a couple of yards. It was called the Great Smog, and it suffocated people and animals. Some 12,000 Londoners died in four days, making it the worst peace-time catastrophe in recent history. As the death toll mounted, undertakers ran out of coffins. The smog was the result of a freak combination of weather factors, emissions from coal-fired factories, and clouds of pollution drifting across the English Channel from Europe. On the fifth day the weather changed and a breeze quickly cleared the air.

The problem with twenty-first-century city pollution is that, unlike the 1952 smog, it isn't easy to see. However, it can be just as dangerous. Children living near busy roads exposed to air pollution are more likely to develop asthma, and they could grow up with reduced lung capacity. Similarly, adults who live in polluted areas are more prone to type 2 diabetes, heart attacks, strokes and cancer.

Recently there have been moves to cut the number of diesel vehicles on British roads, as they are one of the main causes of this pollution – diesel engines produce high levels of particulates and toxic nitrogen oxides. But with a target date of 2040 set as the deadline for phasing out new petrol and diesel vehicles, it is likely to be many years before there is any significant improvement in our air quality.

DR DAWN'S TOP TIP

Many of us have to live or work in towns and cities, or we have to visit places with high air pollution levels. Still, there are a few steps you can take to minimise the risks:

- Avoid unnecessary physical exertion in urban areas and near busy roads.
- If possible, stay inside – concentrations of indoor pollutants are typically a lot lower than in the air outside.
- Install an air filtration system in your home or office – research shows that they can be effective in reducing the levels of harmful chemicals.
- Plan your movements based on pollution forecasts, which are readily available online from the UK Met Office.
- Modify your behaviour based on your personal susceptibility. If you already have asthma or a lung condition such as COPD, you are at much greater risk.

IT'S A DANGEROUS WORLD

In this chapter I have talked about the longevity hotspots, where people tend to live much longer than average. Around the world there are huge variations in life expectancy from one place to another. Depending on where they live, there are many reasons why people die younger than they should.

The WHO regularly compiles a list of the top ten causes of death worldwide. Figure 11.2 gives the latest data, from 2015.

Figure 11.2: Top 10 causes of death globally (2015).

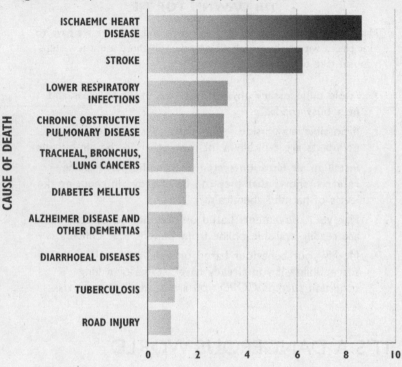

DEATHS IN MILLIONS

These top ten causes explain over half of all the 56.4 million deaths in that year. You can see that heart disease and stroke are by far the biggest killers, accounting for 15 million total deaths. And like any top ten, there are climbers and fallers. Since the last survey (in 2000), deaths from diabetes have gone up from under a million to 1.6 million (see Chapter 4). In the same period deaths from dementia have more than doubled. Meanwhile there has been a big fall in deaths from diarrhoeal diseases and tuberculosis. This is because standards of hygiene and sanitation have improved greatly in many countries.

Nine of the ten causes on the list are health-related. Death from road injury is the exception. We live in a country with one of the world's best road safety records (currently 2.9 deaths per 100,000 of the population per year). So, with a few minor exceptions, every time you leave the UK you are increasing your risk of being killed on the roads. Cross over to France and the death rate almost doubles, to 5.1 deaths per 100,000.

As a general rule, the poorer the country, the higher the road death rate. In Kenya it is 29.1, in Thailand it is 36.2, and at the top of this grim list, with a death rate of 73.4 per 100,000, is Libya.

According to the WHO, only 28 countries worldwide have adequate road safety laws (in that they make provision for speeding, drink-driving, wearing helmets when cycling or motorcycling, using seatbelts or fixing proper child restraints in cars). Half of the 1.3 million road traffic deaths occur among motorcyclists (23%), pedestrians (22%) and cyclists (5%).[10] For people who are otherwise healthy, road traffic accidents are by far the largest cause of death.

DR DAWN'S TOP TIP

If you travel abroad, you should take sensible precautions to reduce the risk of being injured in a road traffic accident:

- Always put children in appropriate car seats.
- When possible, avoid riding in a car at night.
- Don't use motorcycles – but, if you must, wear a helmet, and appropriate clothes.
- Make sure you understand local traffic laws before you drive.
- Only use licensed taxis with seatbelts.
- Avoid overcrowded or top-heavy buses and vans.
- Be alert when crossing the road, particularly in countries where people drive on the right.

These horrendous road death figures tend to get very little publicity, because each accident generally involves a few people and is likely to be in a country where news media are not as extensive or sophisticated as our own. Meanwhile the slightest incident involving an aeroplane makes headline news. Yet the risk involved in flying is infinitesimally small; only one in three million flights ends in a fatal accident. If you travel abroad on holiday, the flight is the safest part of the journey – you are much more likely to be killed in the taxi from the airport to your hotel.

The fear of flying can be much more dangerous than flying itself. In the wake of the 9/11 attacks in America in 2001, huge numbers of Americans were scared of flying and switched to driving long distances instead. Airline passenger miles fell by around 12%. Over the following year the road death toll in the USA increased by 1,595 people.[11] You could say that these people were indirect victims of the terrorist attacks.

As they do with flying, people tend to have extremely inaccurate perceptions of the risks associated with travelling to other countries. So, although these risks are generally very low, here are some other things you might consider before venturing out to visit exotic parts of the globe:

Skiing. Most travel insurance companies will charge you extra if you tell them you intend to go on a skiing holiday – but this is mainly to cover the potentially high cost of sending a helicopter to rescue you from a mountain if you have an accident. For every 1,000 people who go skiing, only three will need any kind of medical treatment. This is really very low – about the same level of risk as for playing a game of football. Furthermore, skiing has been getting less risky in recent years, mainly due to the development of safer equipment.

Sex. You are three times more likely to get a sexually transmitted infection (STI) when you go abroad. This is because travel is associated with much greater risk-taking behaviour. The usual social restraints may be absent, and increased alcohol intake plays a huge part. *Tourism Management* Journal summed it up like this: 'The uniqueness of tourist destinations . . . promotes an altered sense of reality that condones sexual experimentation and exploration while minimising perceptions of risk and long-term consequences.'[12]

Sunshine. Moderate exposure to the sun's rays is beneficial because it boosts the level of vitamin D in your body, but too much can be dangerous. The ultraviolet (UV) light in the sun's rays can cause lasting damage, leading to the risk of skin cancer, including melanoma (see Chapter 8). Having a tan may be considered attractive, but it is actually a visible warning sign that you are putting yourself at risk. Just one episode of sunburn as a child doubles your risk of getting skin cancer as an adult. Exposure to sunshine can also cause premature skin ageing, producing wrinkles and loss of elasticity. So stay in the shade when possible, particularly between 11 a.m. and 3 p.m., when the sun is at its strongest. If you are exposing your skin to the sun, apply generous quantities of a high-factor sunscreen.

Accidents. As well as a generally much higher chance of having a road accident while you're abroad, there is an increased risk of being injured or even killed in accidents of all kinds. Slippery pool sides, loose balcony railings and badly maintained walkways are all potential hazards. Swimming abroad is also associated with greater dangers, whether in unsupervised swimming pools or in the sea.

Murder. As with road accidents, we're lucky to be based in a country where the murder rate is very low (about one person per 100,000 of the population per year). According to the most recent figures from the United Nations, in Jamaica the murder rate is 39.3. In Venezuela it's 53.7, and – topping the homicide list – Honduras's murder rate is 90.4 per 100,000. In recent years Honduras has become increasingly popular as a holiday destination, but tourists are often targeted by criminals in various ways.

Terrorism. Even allowing for all the high-profile attacks in recent years, the risk that you will be killed in any kind of terrorist attack is around 1 in 215,000.[13] That figure includes deaths in places like Iraq and Afghanistan. If you stick to visiting countries that are relatively safe (as advised by the UK government's Foreign and Commonwealth Office), the risk is much lower. President Obama was correct when he said that the chance you will drown in your own bath is considerably higher than your chance of being killed in a terrorist attack.

Foreign diseases. By far the biggest hazard associated with world travel is the risk that you might contract some form of disease that is very rare or even completely unknown in the UK. Illnesses like malaria, typhoid, diphtheria, yellow fever and cholera are hardly ever encountered in the developed world. Poor sanitation can lead to infection with harmful bacteria, particularly in countries where access to clean water is limited. Common ailments can easily be managed in medically advanced countries, but health risks increase significantly in places where the medical infrastructure is inadequate. (See also Chapter 9.)

Pre-existing conditions. If you have a pre-existing health condition such as coronary heart disease, diabetes or high blood pressure, you are statistically much more likely to fall ill while you are on holiday. That's why it's so important to ensure that your travel insurance covers pre-existing conditions. Many people – particularly the elderly – find that it is very expensive, or almost impossible, to get the insurance they need.

DR DAWN'S TOP TIP

Before you travel abroad, I suggest you take the following precautions:

- Always check the government's foreign travel advice website (www.gov.uk/foreign-travel-advice) for the latest information about safety and security, travel warnings and health for every country you are planning to visit.

- Make sure that you and your fellow travellers have suitable travel insurance. This should ensure that you are covered for all the countries you are planning to visit, for any potentially risky activities you may be undertaking (such as skiing), and with explicit provision that you are covered for any problems arising from pre-existing medical conditions.

- About six weeks before you travel anywhere outside Europe, you should schedule an appointment with a nurse or another appropriate healthcare professional to make sure you get the recommended vaccines for those countries. This gives the vaccines enough time to start working; some vaccines may require more than one dose before you go. You can find an up-to-date list of which vaccinations are recommended for any particular country at www.fitfortravel.nhs.uk/destinations.aspx. Some countries won't even let you enter without proof that you've been immunised against certain diseases.

- If you use any medication on a regular basis, make sure you have enough supplies to last you for the duration of your trip. Carry a copy of your prescription for added security. Also, if you are undergoing any special treatment, consider carrying a letter from your doctor that explains your condition.

- If you have a pre-existing medical condition, maybe you should consider limiting your travel aspirations to countries with the highest standards of healthcare. I don't want to be a killjoy, but if you suffer a heart attack in the middle of the Borneo jungle, the chances of your survival will be somewhat lower than if you had gone to Benidorm.

SHOULD YOU EMIGRATE IN ORDER TO LIVE LONGER?

Most people don't have the freedom to live where they would really like to live. As we get older we become locked into lifestyle patterns based on where we work, where we can afford to live, or where we send our children to school. As we get older still, we often find that family ties become the main limitation on our options when choosing a home.

Many people move to the seaside or to a foreign country to enjoy better weather in their later years, but a large percentage regret doing so because they miss their friends, relatives or familiar places. Although a high percentage of people (57% in a recent survey[14]) say they would like to retire abroad, only about 8,000 British people actually do so every year – that's less than 1%.

Having spent four days in Acciaroli, I can easily see the appeal. There's fresh sea air, plenty of sunshine and readily available supplies of healthy Mediterranean food. I'll let Acciaroli's mayor, Stefano Pisani, have the last word: 'Who wouldn't want to live in a beautiful place like this? There's very little crime and the people are friendly. And if you do get homesick, you can always go up to Naples and fly back to the UK!'

CHAPTER 12
MONEY MATTERS

Imagine that you could afford to hire leading private doctors and specialists to be on call at short notice at any time of the day or night, so that every minor health problem you might experience gets immediate attention. Imagine that each time you go abroad you take a doctor with you, as well as an emergency supply of blood. And imagine that you could get comprehensive health checks on a regular basis to detect potentially serious conditions at an early stage.

Well, this is what the senior members of the British Royal Family enjoy. The Royals seem to have an outstanding ability to live long (and reasonably healthy) lives. Part of this longevity may be down to genetics. But to what extent does money play a part?

The Queen has become the longest-serving monarch in British history. To date she has seen twelve prime ministers come and go, and she has outlived many of her subjects. She has access to a team of doctors called the Medical Household, the head of which is known by the grand title of Apothecary to Her Majesty and the Royal Household. She has regular health checks, as well as annual medical screenings at London's King Edward VII Hospital. When she travels, she typically has the support of over 30 staff who will monitor every detail of her itinerary, including what she eats and whether hygienic lavatories are available at every location. On these occasions her Royal Navy doctor is never more than a few paces away, carrying not only packs of blood but also a mobile defibrillator and all manner of emergency medicine.

Although the Queen's medical history is of course secret, we do know a bit about her past ailments. She had a wisdom tooth removed in 1982, and she needed stitches in her hand after being bitten by one of her corgis in 1993. In 2013 she was admitted to hospital for a suspected case of gastroenteritis. But by any standards her health seems remarkably good.

Other members of the Royal Family have also achieved lifespans that are far above average, such as the Queen Mother, who lived to the age of 101. Most British monarchs have lived longer than their life expectancy at birth – the only exception in recent times has been George VI, the Queen's father, who was a heavy smoker and who died of lung cancer at the age of 56 as a direct result. King George III and Queen Victoria both lived to the age of 81. Going much further back (to the year 1307) we find that King Edward I lived to 68 at a time when the average male life expectancy was just 40.

So it's normal for our monarchs to outlive the average person. If you could afford a similar lifestyle, would that sort of extreme wealth and privilege also give you a much better shot at living to a healthy old age?

THE WEALTH GAP

Take another look at the life expectancy figures given in Chapter 1. One thing is very obvious: people in wealthy countries generally live a lot longer than those in poor countries. Citizens of Japan, Switzerland, Australia and France are living on average into their eighties while residents of Sierra Leone, Lesotho and the Central African Republic are lucky if they make it to 50. There are some exceptions to this pattern: in Bangladesh and Nepal, life expectancies are in the mid-60s, even though these are poor countries. And some rich countries do much worse than their wealth would suggest. The

USA is an example: it has the world's largest economy, but only comes in at number 43 in the life expectancy league table. Americans die younger than people in almost every other wealthy country. This may be because they are more likely to have alcohol and drug problems and, because of the widespread possession of guns, they suffer far more violent deaths compared to their peer countries: in 2013, there were 33,636 firearms deaths in the USA.[1] Also, because on average they consume more calories than anyone else, people in the USA also have the highest rate of type 2 diabetes and one of the highest rates of heart disease.

When we look at what's happening in the UK, we find that the gap in life expectancy between rich and poor is large – and it's getting bigger. Recent figures show that the richest 5% of British men live on average to 96.2 years – 34.2 years longer than the poorest 10%. The richest women achieve an average age of 98.5 years, 31.5 years older than the poorest. According to the Cass Business School (City, University of London), this gap is wider than it was 20 years ago.[2] This is not because life expectancies have fallen; they've gone up for everyone. It's just that the rich have pulled ahead and are living disproportionately longer.

Consider these figures for a moment. These age differences are huge – not just a year or two, but the equivalent of the rich living 50% longer than their poorest compatriots. At first glance, it doesn't seem very fair. But what are the real reasons for this gap? Does the simple fact of having money do anything to benefit your health? Well, in one way it does, because richer people tend to be happier and (as we saw in Chapter 10) happiness is closely linked to life expectancy.

The link between money and happiness was measured in a huge study carried out by two leading economists, Betsey Stevenson and Justin Wolfers[3] based on interviews with hundreds of thousands of people in 166 countries. They found that people in richer countries were more satisfied with their lives than people in poorer countries.

Within each country, richer people also described themselves as being happier than those with lower incomes. It seems that if you double your income you gain about half a point on a '1 to 10' scale of life satisfaction.

In other respects, having money doesn't necessarily make a huge difference. I like this quote from Bill Gates (of Microsoft fame), who has at various times been the world's richest man: 'I can understand wanting to have millions of dollars . . . but once you get beyond that, I have to tell you it's the same hamburger.'[4]

Rich people do tend to have other advantages: for example, they are likely to have much lower levels of work-related stress. They are more likely to be business owners or high achievers who are not answerable to someone else. If they do get ill, they can take time off to recover. Many very rich people do not work at all because they don't need to. And when they do have medical problems, they don't have to take their chance with the National Health Service; they can pay to see a private doctor.

PRIVATE HEALTHCARE

There are many reasons why people choose to 'go private'. It may be to get faster treatment or to access procedures that are not readily available on the NHS (such as certain types of cosmetic surgery). For many people private healthcare means the added comfort of having a pleasant room in a modern hospital with better food. You can get private health treatment for almost any medical condition, including dental treatment, physiotherapy, counselling and psychotherapy, or treatment for drug or alcohol abuse.

About 80% of people who get private treatment rely on medical insurance to pay for it, either funded by themselves or by their employer. But the NHS often contracts out treatments to private hospitals and clinics, so you could get the benefits without having to pay.

DR DAWN'S TOP TIP

If you do decide to get private medical treatment, make sure you find out exactly what it will cost in advance. Will there be extra charges for unforeseen events and complications? If you are relying on health insurance, make sure the treatment you are having is covered by your insurance policy. From my experience, there's a lot of 'small print' in insurers' terms and conditions, and they will often try to find a way to wriggle out of paying for what seems like a perfectly reasonable medical procedure.

So whether you actually pay or not, is private medicine better than NHS healthcare? We have all seen horrendous stories in the news about things going wrong in NHS hospitals, but since the public sector accounts for the vast majority of treatments, this is as you would expect. The NHS is one of the most transparent healthcare systems in the world, publishing large amounts of data about every hospital and consultant. In my experience, private treatment also results in frequent claims for clinical negligence, although these occurrences tend to get less publicity. Whether you go private or use the NHS, there's always a small risk of a poor outcome with any medical procedure.

In a survey of patients carried out in 2015,[5] 79% of the British public said they would prefer to use the NHS if they needed emergency treatment. That's not surprising – for a start, most people simply wouldn't have the option of going private, and Accident & Emergency departments don't exist as such in the private sector.

I can't tell you whether or not to go private (if you or your employer can afford it). You will get quicker access to treatment, but the eventual outcome may be much the same as if you had gone with the NHS.

The one area where private medicine does consistently seem to have the edge is in dealing with so-called hospital-acquired infections. Hospital 'superbugs' such as MRSA and *C. difficile* are a serious problem in a large number of NHS hospitals, causing deaths, or forcing many patients to have a longer hospital stay. In the worst cases they can cause permanent disability or even death.

In private hospitals such infections are much easier to control, partly because patients have their own rooms, but also because the staff-to-patient ratio tends to be higher, and there are also more cleaners. Several private hospitals in the UK have been able to boast that they have had no cases of MRSA at all.

CHECK UP ON HEALTH CHECKS

Baroness Karren Brady is a well-known British entrepreneur. She made her name as a sporting executive, as managing director of Birmingham City, and subsequently as vice-chairman of West Ham United. But she is perhaps best known to the British public for being one of Lord Sugar's aides on the BBC TV series *The Apprentice*.

When she was 36, Karren booked a private medical health screen, which included a full-body MRI scan. The scan showed that she had a cerebral aneurysm, a weakened artery in the brain that put her at risk of having a haemorrhage or a stroke. It could have ruptured and killed her at any moment. One doctor expressed surprise that she had managed to survive giving birth to her two children. She was told she needed to see a specialist immediately.

Faced with a variety of surgical options, Karren decided to have a coil implanted inside her brain to seal the aneurysm from its blood supply. This 'coiling' involved inserting a fine catheter through an artery in her groin, an operation that took five hours and which was followed by 24 hours in intensive care. She was then off work for a further six weeks.

Now, several years later, she still has to have regular check-ups but she is convinced that the scan saved her life. 'My doctor says the results are as good as they could be. The swelling on the artery has

sealed up. But being faced with this made me realise how lucky I am,'
she said. 'I woke up and realised that I really love my life and want
to live it as long as possible' (Stacey, S. (2013) 'Health Notes: Karren
Brady on life after a stroke, relief for kids from chicken pox and
relieving facial tension', *Mail on Sunday*[6]).

Karren now also works for the Stroke Association, a leading
charity that aims to raise awareness of the dangers of having a stroke.

This is indeed a cautionary tale. Should we all have regular scans
and check-ups to catch the early signs of potentially fatal conditions?
It helps if you have money. The clinic where Karren Brady had her
scan currently charges £3,600 for its 'Ultimate' check-up, and a few
hundred pounds more if you want the 'Ultimate Plus'. Irrespective of
the cost, are these scans and tests a good idea?

Even though there are many cases in which a health check has
probably saved someone's life, they are controversial. For a start, they
don't always pick up potentially serious conditions, and there is also
the problem of 'false positives' (where the diagnosis of a medical
problem later turns out to be wrong). In these cases, people may
have treatment they didn't actually need (see Chapter 8).

In 2009 the NHS started to offer free checks at GP surgeries to
everyone aged between 40 and 74. You can have a test every five
years. It includes checks on blood pressure and cholesterol, as well as
looking for indicators that could be linked to the possibility of
diabetes, kidney problems or a potential stroke.

The NHS health check addresses nine of the seventeen risk
factors for cardiovascular disease. Since this is the greatest cause of
premature death in the UK (see Chapter 7), anything that helps us
identify the risks and do something about them before it's too late
has got to be a good thing. If you're over 65 you'll also be checked
for signs of dementia. In terms of preventing medical problems,
however, it seems the results have been disappointing. That's mainly
because only one in five adults in the target age group have actually
made an appointment to have their 'mid-life MOT'.

DR DAWN'S TOP TIP

If you're invited for your NHS health check, don't ignore the invitation. The appointment should be a priority, and it could save your life. If you haven't been invited for a few years, contact your GP surgery to find out whether you may be eligible for a free check.

If you don't mind paying for health checks, there's a wide variety of options. I've already mentioned genetic tests (see Chapter 2), which can cost hundreds or even thousands of pounds. But if you're feeling rich, here are some others you might consider:

Private health assessment: Many clinics and health insurers offer a comprehensive package of health tests to identify potential problems. A typical test will last up to three hours, and will include a detailed physical examination by a doctor, blood and urine tests, as well as an assessment of your physical fitness. Some places will also include a sight and hearing test. The test will also be slightly different for men and women, to detect early signs of gender-specific cancers. Expect to pay anywhere between £200 and £2,000, depending on the extent of the test (and how posh the clinic looks!).

MRI scan: This stands for magnetic resonance imaging, a process whereby magnetic fields and radio waves are used to produce detailed images of your body. During the scan you have to lie completely still on a horizontal surface. MRI is used to examine the brain, spinal cord, internal organs, joints, bones, heart and blood vessels. The scan takes from about ten minutes up to an hour or more, and you could expect to pay around a few hundred pounds per body part or area, or (as already mentioned) much more if it's part of a more comprehensive health assessment.

CT scan: An alternative to MRI, a CT scan (also called a CAT scan) uses X-rays to look at the organs inside your body.

You may need to drink a 'contrast agent' a few hours beforehand: this is a chalky-tasting liquid that enhances the structures and fluids in the body to make the resulting images clearer. The scan usually takes up to ten minutes, and you would expect to pay several hundred pounds. Because a CT scan uses radiation, it is not suitable for young children or pregnant women.

Ultrasound scan: In an ultrasound, high-frequency sound waves are used to produce an image of the tissues inside your body. Unlike CT, ultrasound is completely safe, which is why it's used to check on developing babies in pregnant women. Rather than scanning your whole body, these tests tend to be used to examine part of you, such as your liver, kidney, urinary tract, heart, thyroid and neck, pelvis, groin, etc. Each scan would normally cost about £100–£200.

DR DAWN'S TOP TIP

It is a legal requirement that all providers of screening services in the UK are registered with the Care Quality Commission. Before you book anything, check that they are listed (cqc.org.uk) and, if possible, do some further research to find out whether they have a good reputation. Before any test, you should ask for clear information about the risks involved as well as the potential benefits.

Screening is not the right option for people with existing symptoms. If you are worried about your health and you are experiencing symptoms you should visit your GP. Before you pay for any sort of test or scan, you should find out whether it is available on the NHS. You may need a doctor's referral, but in many cases you may find that you can have the test for free.

You should also remember that most private health screening companies do not offer a full medical service so, if a problem is detected, you will need to look elsewhere for the care and treatment you may need.

Although the number of people going for expensive full-body scans is relatively small, in another area of medical check-ups there is currently a boom. Home testing kits first appeared in the 1970s when pregnancy tests went on sale in high-street chemists. Now you can also buy tests for HIV, colon cancer, hepatitis C, urinary tract infections, diabetes, Alzheimer's, prostate cancer, stomach ulcers and any number of other potentially serious medical conditions. In the UK the market for these tests is estimated to be worth around £60 million a year, with the various tests either being sold in shops or (more commonly) on the internet.

People like these tests because they are convenient – a quick, simple test in the comfort of your own home means you can avoid making a trip to see your GP. They are also private, so no one else needs to know you're taking a test – or its outcome. But home testing kits have limitations: they can be difficult to use and can be unreliable, resulting in false alarms or false reassurance.

DR DAWN'S TOP TIP

If you are tempted to use a home testing medical kit, you are probably wiser (and certainly better off) going straight to your GP, who would in any case have to carry out further tests to confirm any findings made by such kits.

HEALTHY, WEALTHY AND WISE

So, can you buy your way to a longer life? We would have to conduct some sort of social experiment to find out. For example, we could look at the lifespans of lottery winners. People who play the UK's National Lottery tend to come from homes with below-average incomes. Once they've won a jackpot (say over £1,000,000) they are immediately propelled into the top 2% of richest people in the country. So, statistically, we would expect them to live longer –

maybe a lot longer, if their lottery win happened while they were still young. But as the first lottery draw was in 1994, the vast majority of people who participate are alive anyway, irrespective of whether or not they've won a jackpot. We'll need to wait another 50 years before we can see if there's a pattern.[7]

There is some evidence that improved wealth can lead to improved health, and it comes from a village in Surrey. Whiteley Village is a charitable community near Walton-on-Thames. It was founded around a century ago with a £1 million bequest from the founder of Whiteleys department store in Bayswater, west London. Today it describes itself as a 'charitable retirement community supporting older people of limited means to live as independently as possible'.

The village is an attractive cluster of picture-postcard almshouses with a shop and pub, set in over 200 acres of wooded countryside. Based on the terms of the original Whiteley request, in order to receive a place, you must be an 'aged poor person'. The decision about who gets in is made by the charitable trust that runs the village. Ironically, Whiteley Village is within walking distance of St George's Hill, Weybridge, one of the wealthiest private estates in the UK.

Whiteley Village is notable for its number of elderly residents. While it may not be as remarkable as Acciaroli in Italy (see Chapter 11), at present it has 11 centenarians and many more inhabitants who are well into their nineties.

An organisation called the International Longevity Centre UK has conducted research into the lifespans of Whiteley Village residents. They analysed the records of 2,614 residents who had lived there since its foundation in 1917. They found that women who moved there in retirement could expect, on average, an extra five years of life. The gains in longevity have been recorded over several decades in women from the poorest 20% of the population, who would usually be expected to die earlier than average. Although men have fared less well, this evidence suggests that you can significantly boost the prospects for an 'aged poor person' by giving them a better standard of living than they could otherwise have afforded.

So if you're poor or 'just about managing' on an average income, are the longevity dice stacked against you? I don't think they are. Although the lifespan 'wealth gap' between the very richest and the very poorest is huge, this is probably not a simple case of cause and effect.

As I mentioned earlier, the clinical outcomes for people receiving private treatment are not generally that much better than for those on the NHS. And although health scans can save lives, not everyone believes they are a good thing.

It probably comes down to the type of person you are. I think it's fair to say that rich people seem to place greater store on looking after themselves. Through good diet and plenty of exercise they can significantly reduce the risks of getting potentially fatal diseases.

In contrast, poor people are more likely to make damaging lifestyle choices. Professor Les Mayhew of Cass Business School at the City, University of London (whose research produced the lifespan figures at the start of this chapter) puts it like this: 'They smoke more, they drink more, and there are periods in their lives when they do crazy things. They are also more likely to be obese, take less exercise and eat an unhealthy diet.'[8]

Of course, there are many deep-seated psychological reasons for over-eating, drinking too much, smoking, or taking drugs. Some of these are explored at https://www.psychologytoday.com/blog/compassion-matters/201205/whats-behind-emotional-overeating. If you feel you have psychological problems around eating, do make an appointment to see your GP. Counselling may help to resolve such issues.

To summarise, the people who take care of themselves and follow all my 'top tips' to stay healthy are those who are generally more motivated to make positive lifestyle choices. And, because they're more motivated, proactive and dynamic, they're more likely to be successful and become rich!

You could follow their example and live well to 101 – and have the added benefit of making lots of money along the way.

CHAPTER 13

THE ELIXIR
OF LIFE

Nobody's perfect. We all have weaknesses. Good intentions only go so far. I'm not expecting anyone to completely change their lifestyle as a result of reading this book. But even a few small changes here or there could make a big difference to how healthy you are and how long you're likely to live.

In terms of longevity, you can make a reasonable guess about what to expect. Table 13.1 shows the latest figures from the Office of National Statistics for average lifespans in the UK (rounded up or down to the nearest whole year). As you can see, when you're born you could expect to live to 79 if you're male, and 83 if you're female. These figures stay much the same until you reach the age of 35–40. Then they start going up: because you've managed to survive that far, your chances of having a longer life increase. If you actually make it to the average age of death, you can then expect a further nine years if you're a man, or eight years if you're a woman. Even when you get to the age of 100, you can still expect on average a couple more years on earth.

You can then adjust your predicted life expectancy based on your personal health or lifestyle. There are – of course – lots of variables, and they will differ depending on how old you are right now. But here's what happens when you apply some of these factors to the prospects for a 40-year-old woman:

Smoking. If you're a heavy smoker or you've smoked reasonably heavily throughout your adult life, deduct 10 years. (Obviously this would be less if you smoke less, but it's still pretty frightening.)

Alcohol. If you're a heavy drinker (defined as drinking over 21 units a week), take off 8 years.

Exercise. If you take lots of exercise on a regular basis, you can add 4 years.

Cardiovascular disease. If this was the cause of death for a close relative who died before they were 50, deduct 2 years. If that person was over 50, deduct 1 year.

Genes. If both your parents lived to over 75, add 4 years.

Weight. If you're obese, deduct 6 years. If you're morbidly obese, deduct 9 years.

Diet. If you eat the recommended five portions a day of fruit or vegetables, add 2 years.

Relationship. If you're happily married or in a similarly stable relationship, add 2 years. If you have an active social life with a good network of friends, add 4 years.

Mood. If you're a happy and optimistic person, add 2 years. If you would describe yourself as unhappy or depressed, deduct 2 years.

You get the idea. Most insurance companies make a risk assessment of each new applicant based on factors such as these. If you want a more detailed idea of your own personal prognosis, I suggest you try one of these online life expectancy calculators:

Confused.com – www.confused.com/life-insurance/life-expectancy-calculator

SunLife – www.sunlife.co.uk/life-cover/over-50-life-insurance/death-clock/

My Key Man Insurance – www.mykeymaninsurance.com/life-expectancy-calculator/

Table 13.1: Average life expectancies in the UK.

Age now	Male	female	Age now	Male	female	Age now	Male	female
0	79	83	36	80	84	72	85	87
1	79	83	37	80	84	73	86	87
2	79	83	38	80	84	74	86	88
3	79	83	39	80	84	75	86	88
4	79	83	40	80	84	76	87	88
5	79	83	41	80	84	77	87	89
6	79	83	42	81	84	78	87	89
7	79	83	43	81	84	79	88	89
8	79	83	44	81	84	80	88	90
9	79	83	45	81	84	81	89	90
10	79	83	46	81	84	82	89	90
11	80	83	47	81	84	83	90	91
12	80	83	48	81	84	84	90	91
13	80	83	49	81	84	85	91	92
14	80	83	50	81	84	86	91	92
15	80	83	51	81	84	87	92	93
16	80	83	52	81	84	88	93	93
17	80	83	53	81	84	89	93	94
18	80	83	54	82	85	90	94	95
19	80	83	55	82	85	91	95	95
20	80	83	56	82	85	92	95	96
21	80	83	57	82	85	93	96	97
22	80	83	58	82	85	94	97	97
23	80	83	59	82	85	95	98	98
24	80	83	60	82	85	96	99	99
25	80	83	61	83	85	97	99	100
26	80	83	62	83	85	98	100	101
27	80	83	63	83	86	99	101	101
28	80	83	64	83	86	100	102	102
29	80	83	65	83	86	101	103	103
30	80	83	66	84	86	102	104	104
31	80	83	67	84	86	103	105	105
32	80	83	68	84	86	104	106	106
33	80	83	69	84	87	105	107	107
34	80	83	70	85	87	106	107	108
35	80	84	71	85	87	107	108	109

AGE IS JUST A NUMBER

When I started writing this book, I had a very open mind about what my core message would be. I knew it would involve healthy eating, but I really wanted to take on board the things I've heard from the amazing centenarians I have met while doing research. They come from very different backgrounds, but whether it is Ann Baer from London or Giuseppe Vassallo from the beautiful Italian town of Acciaroli, they have some very striking things in common.

All the centenarians who were generous enough to talk openly to me about their lives have had quite hard childhoods by modern standards. They were of course children in pre-motorcar days, so they walked everywhere. They were simply more active. Today, those of us who are interested in keeping fit put aside time each week to exercise, but because of the way we lead our lives, the rest of our week is often relatively sedentary.

It also struck me that every single person I interviewed eats a lot of fish. Jimmy Thirsk from Kent was keen to tell me that, at the age of 102, he catches the bus into town each week to buy fresh fish, which he cooks for himself. And, along with fish, all the centenarians I met eat a lot of fresh vegetables. Their cooking may be relatively simple, but they all enjoy a variety of seasonal veg. I have certainly increased my fish and vegetable intake since meeting these wonderful people.

Finally, they all have a very positive attitude to life. I think of Jock Stares from South Wales. He was utterly heartbroken when his wife Babs died 16 years ago. He told me he was a total misery and then one evening he wrote a letter to himself telling him to be grateful for the years he had spent with her, and to make the most of whatever time he had left. The following morning he read his letter and took his own advice. He got on his motorbike, drove to a local nursing home and played the piano to the residents. I was privileged to visit Jock in his home and hear his piano playing. He is a very accomplished pianist and played me old wartime songs that really made me smile. I am sure he must be a real tonic to the residents of the nursing homes he visits. Today, he keeps busy by visiting a different care home each day. He has such a wonderfully positive and generous attitude to life, and this is a common theme in all the centenarians I have met – they continue to live life to the full. They also have a total disdain for stress! Jimmy finds peace and fulfilment in his living room lined with books, Giuseppe passes the day playing cards with his friends in the Mediterranean sun – they simply don't allow themselves to succumb to stress.

You may argue that it is easy to avoid stress when you are no longer working and when you have been retired for years, but as I talked to these people it became abundantly clear that they had never allowed themselves to get stressed.

In summary, here are my five top tips for healthy longevity:

1. **Be active.** Keep up your formal activity (exercise classes and so on), but take a step back and look at your week to find ways in which you could be more active. It may be something as simple as putting your printer in a different room so you have to walk to collect printouts!

2. **Eat more fish.** The people I interviewed are testimony to the benefits of a pescatarian diet.

3. **Eat a variety of vegetables.** I am increasingly convinced of the benefits of aiming for at least five portions of vegetables per day. Your plate should look like a rainbow of colour.

4. **Think positively and manage your stress.** Do something each day to make those around you smile. Managing stress is easier said than done, but there will be something each one of us can do to reduce our stress. Working out what this is will be time well invested.

5. **Keep in touch with friends and family**. Make an effort to
   get out and join in – every single one of the active
   centenarians I met was still an active part of their community.

I started this book by promising that my tips on how to live well
into old age would be easily achievable. I hope you agree that
nothing in this book is difficult – it just takes a bit of planning, but it's
well worth doing.

Now, it just remains for me to wish you long life and good health!

CHAPTER 14
AND FINALLY . . .

I have based everything I have written so far in this book on a combination of my own medical experience, meetings with various centenarians, and research into healthy living and longevity. However, while writing, I came across some other theories that are worth a mention. They may not be supported by the most rigorous gerontological science, but they are at least entertaining. I'll leave it up to you to decide whether they could be effective.

EAT SPICY FOOD

Hot curries could – literally – be the spice of life. The Chinese Academy of Medical Sciences carried out a survey[1] of the eating habits of 487,000 people aged from 30 to 80. They found that people who ate vindaloo, madras or jalfrezi dishes once or twice a week were 10% less likely to die than a comparable group of people who did not eat curries. Better still, those who ate three or more curries a week had a reduced mortality rate of 14%. They said the curry eaters were less likely to die, even if they already had diabetes, cancer or heart disease. Dr Nita Forouhi from the University of Cambridge reviewed the results. Her conclusion? 'More research is needed.'

FOLLOW YOUR NOSE

Your sense of smell could predict your lifespan. Researchers from the University of Chicago asked a representative sample of people aged from 57 to 85 to take part in a smell test. They were asked to identify five odours – peppermint, fish, orange, rose and leather. Five years later, 39% of the people with the lowest scores (4–5 errors) had died, compared with just 10% of those with a healthy sense of smell (0–1 error). The researchers made allowance for other factors, such as age, nutrition, smoking habits and overall health. The university's Professor Jayant Pinto said: 'We think loss of the sense of smell is like the canary in the coal mine. It doesn't directly cause death, but it is a harbinger, an early warning system that shows damage may have been done. [It's] a quick, inexpensive way to identify patients most at risk.'[2]

CAERPHILLY DOES IT

This is another food-based theory – this time from Aarhus University in Denmark. Their 2015 study[3] concluded that eating aged cheeses such as Brie, Parmesan and Cheddar could add years to your life. In particular, they compared the diets of British and French people. The French enjoy a low incidence of coronary heart disease and an average life expectancy of 82 years (while eating 23.9kg of cheese per person per year). We British eat just 11.6kg of cheese each year: our life expectancy is about a year less, and we have much higher levels of cardiovascular disease. The researchers say cheese contains a substance called butyric acid, which has been linked to reduced obesity and higher metabolism. Another study[4] singled out Roquefort cheese as being particularly beneficial.

SMILES BETTER

Whether or not you like eating cheese, just saying the word could do wonders. Next time someone asks you to smile for the camera, it might be wise to heed their advice. Researchers at Wayne State University in Michigan, USA,[5] studied team photos of former professional Major League baseball players and found that, the bigger their smile, the longer they lived. They explained: 'Facial expressions are a barometer of the emotions. Smile intensity [is] correlated with marriage stability and satisfaction.' Of the baseball players who had died at the time of the study, players with no smiles lived an average of 72.9 years, while those with big, authentic-looking grins lived an average of 79.9 years. Living an extra seven years certainly seems like something to smile about.

THE RIGHT STUFF

OK, so this is one you can't do much to change. In 1988 the journal *Nature*[6] published research suggesting that right-handed people live an average of nine years longer than left-handed people. This was partly because, in a world designed for right-handers, left-handers tend to have more accidents. A further American study in 2001[7] came to the same conclusion, but with a reduced longevity advantage of only 3.7 years for right-handers. About 10% of the world's population is left-handed. Not surprisingly, these findings have been very controversial; more recent research suggests that this left/right longevity gap is probably a myth.

FEEL THE HEAT

A study of men in Finland (where else?)[8] suggests that taking
frequent saunas helps you live longer. The study tracked around
2,000 men for 20 years. Those who took the most saunas (4–7
times a week) had half the rate of deaths from heart attacks and
strokes. Overall the men in this group had a 40% reduction in their
risk of dying from any cause. The theory is that a sauna gives your
body a shock of heat, which can activate a 'longevity gene' known as
FOX03. This in turn promotes the production of disease-fighting
antioxidants, maintenance of proteins, and repair of your DNA.

GO GREEN

The trees, shrubs and plants outside your home might offer
something more than just pretty scenery. A team from the Harvard
T.H. Chan School of Public Health in Boston, USA, found that
women who live in or near green areas live longer and have
improved mental health.[9] The study tracked 108,000 women over an
eight-year period and measured the amount of vegetation near their
homes using satellite imagery. The women living in the greenest areas
had a 12% lower death rate than those living in the least green
areas. Most lived in urban areas. It's not necessary to move to the
countryside; simply planting lots of trees and bushes near your home
seems to have a beneficial effect. The research team concluded that
people who live in greener areas have increased opportunities for
social engagement, a higher level of physical activity and lower
exposure to air pollution.

READ ALL ABOUT IT

Being an avid reader can add around two years to your life. A 2016 study published in *Social Science & Medicine* journal[10] divided people into three groups: those who read no books, those who read books for up to 3.5 hours a week, and those who read books for over 3.5 hours a week. They made allowances for other factors such as state of health, age and lifestyle. Compared to those who did not read books, those who read the most were 23% less likely to die over the following 12 years. The researchers found a similar association among those who read newspapers and magazines, but it was weaker. So, if you've enjoyed this book, why not find yourself a comfortable sofa, lie back, relax and read it again?

ACKNOWLEDGEMENTS

I would like to thank my agent Debbie for her unwavering encouragement and support; Lindsey Evans, Kate Miles, Jane Hammett, Siobhan Hooper, Phoebe Swinburn, Viviane Basset, Louise Rothwell and the team at Headline Home and Julian and Ben at LAW for believing in this project from day one; all my wonderful patients and the centenarians I have met while writing this book, who really bring the concept to life; Victor van Amerongen for his extensive research; and my lovely better half Jack, for holding the fort at home while I spent hours researching and writing.

NOTES

(All websites accessed in August 2017.)

CHAPTER I

1. http://journals.plos.org/plosbiology/article?id=10.1371/journal.pbio.0020012

2. https://www.amazon.co.uk/How-Why-Age-Leonard-Hayflick/dp/0345401557

3. http://user.demogr.mpg.de/jwv/pdf/sciencemay2002.pdf

4. http://discovermagazine.com/2009/new-science-of-health/23-modest-proposal-how-to-stop-aging-entirely

5. https://motherboard.vice.com/en_us/article/mgbb9v/meet-aubrey-de-grey-the-researcher-who-wants-to-cure-old-age

6. www.bbc.com/future/story/20140821-i-will-be-frozen-when-i-die

7. www.bbc.com/future/story/20140821-i-will-be-frozen-when-i-die

8. www.elsa-project.ac.uk/uploads/elsa/report06/ch11.pdf

9. www.bbc.co.uk/radio4/reith2001/survey.shtml

10. www.pewforum.org/2013/08/06/living-to-120-and-beyond-americans-views-on-aging-medical-advances-and-radical-life-extension/

11. www.kcl.ac.uk/ioppn/news/records/2015/July/Researchersmeasureageingprocessinyoungadults.aspx

12. http://www.telegraph.co.uk/news/science/science-news/11721228/Why-you-might-be-20-years-older-than-your-actual-age.html

13. For example, www.biological-age.com/, http://growyouthful.com/gettestinfo.php?testtype=quizb, http://pinetribe.com/thorbjorg/age-test/ and www.health.com/health/article/0,,20824577,00.html

14. www.thelancet.com/journals/lancet/article/PIIS0140-6736(15)60175-1/fulltext

CHAPTER 2

1. http://www.bbc.com/news/magazine-19648992

2. www.nytimes.com/2013/05/14/opinion/my-medical-choice.html?hp and www.dailymail.co.uk/health/article-3252402/Angelina-Jolie-effect-real-Actress-double-mastectomy-reconstruction-raised-awareness-cancer-treatment.html

3. www.ncbi.nlm.nih.gov/pubmed/25510853 and www.nhs.uk/Conditions/predictive-genetic-tests-cancer/Pages/Introduction.aspx

4. www.thesun.co.uk/archives/health/271207/how-death-of-sir-david-frosts-son-aged-just-31-could-help-save-120000-people/

5. www.livescience.com/53157-genes-centenarians.html

6. http://newsroom.ucla.edu/releases/epigenetic-clock-predicts-life-expectancy-ucla-led-study-shows

7. www.ncbi.nlm.nih.gov/pubmed/11872902 (and see also www.researchgate.net/publication/8514597_The_Danish_Twin_Registry_Past_and_Present for more information on this study)

8. www.nejm.org/doi/full/10.1056/NEJM199404143301503#t=article

9. http://www.telegraph.co.uk/science/2017/01/19/four-10-british-mothers-drink-pregnancy-one-worst-rates-europe/

10. www.independent.co.uk/news/elixir-of-youth-tested-successfully-on-mice-next-for-humans

11. www.wired.com/2009/03/designerdebate/

12. Kolata, G. (2006), 'Live long? Die young? Answer Isn't Just in genes.' At www.nytimes.com/2006/08/31/health/31age.html

CHAPTER 3

1. https://academic.oup.com/aje/article/156/3/268/71617/Environmental-Tobacco-Smoke-and-Risk-of-Malignant

2. Ott, W., Langan, L. and Switzer, P. (1992) 'A time series model for cigarette smoking activity patterns: model validation for carbon monoxide and respirable particles in a chamber and an automobile.' *Journal of Exposure Analysis and Environmental Epidemiology*, 2(2): 175–200.

3. www.nhs.uk/livewell/smoking/Pages/stopsmokingnewhome.aspx

CHAPTER 4

1. www.nhs.uk/Livewell/loseweight/Pages/statistics-and-causes-of-the-obesity-epidemic-in-the-uk.aspx

2. Speech by Dame Sally Davies at the Childhood Obesity Summit, 2017. See https://www.theguardian.com/society/2016/nov/03/chief-medical-officer-obesity-school-warning-letters-parents

CHAPTER 5

1. www.bhf.org.uk/heart-matters-magazine/nutrition/5-a-day/colourful-foods

2. www.gov.uk/government/collections/national-diet-and-nutrition-survey

3. www.nhs.uk/Livewell/Goodfood/Pages/red-meat.aspx

4. For more on vitamin A, see www.niams.nih.gov/Health_Info/Bone/Bone_Health/Nutrition/vitamin_a.asp

CHAPTER 6

1. www.emeraldinsight.com/doi/abs/10.1108/17538350810926534

2. http://time.com/4475628/the-new-science-of-exercise/

3. https://link.springer.com/article/10.1007/BF03340126

4. www.ncbi.nlm.nih.gov/pubmed/21618162

5. https://academic.oup.com/aje/article/172/4/419/85345/Leisure-Time-Spent-Sitting-in-Relation-to-Total

6. http://journals.plos.org/plosmedicine/article?id=10.1371/journal.pmed.1001917

7. www.planningforcare.co.uk/tag/british/

8. https://www.cyclinguk.org/article/campaigns-guide/cycling-levels-in-european-countries

9. http://www.bmj.com/content/348/bmj.g2219

10. http://calorielab.com/burned/?mo=se&gr=15&ti=sports&q=&wt=150&un=lb&kg=68

11. www.lboro.ac.uk/news-events/news/2017/january/weekend-warriors-fight-off-death-for-longer.html

12. https://www.st-andrews.ac.uk/media/capod/staff/wellbeing/documents/step_on_it_article.pdf

13. https://www.gov.uk/government/news/6-million-adults-do-not-do-a-monthly-brisk-10-minute-walk

14. www.nhs.uk/oneyou/active10/home#V2LjK8xLPmal6upg.97

15. www.eiseverywhere.com/ereg/popups/speakerdetails.php?eventid=52907&language=eng&speakerid=171257&

16. www.theargus.co.uk/news/14163029.Dancing_burns_more_calories_than_running___and_makes_you_happier/

CHAPTER 7

1. www.dementiacarecentral.com/aboutdementia/facts/stages/

CHAPTER 8

1. www.ncbi.nlm.nih.gov/pmc/articles/PMC2659709/

CHAPTER 10

1. www.telegraph.co.uk/news/health/news/9323562/We-are-more-likely-to-die-on-our-birthday-than-any-other-day.html

2. www.ucl.ac.uk/news/news-articles/0114/21012014-Enjoying-life-keeps-you-healthy-Steptoe

3. www.dailymail.co.uk/health/article-2980770/It-s-true-Optimists-live-longer-Having-positive-attitude-lowers-risk-heart-attack.html

4. https://books.google.co.uk/s?id=Qbz9NfYdg6UC&pg=PA153&lpg=PA153&dq=%22william+farr%22+%22wrecked+on+his+voyage%22&source=bl&ots=ft_dpp0EIt&sig=EHif6VX3HJ2_3Pw_yVPyBKbTlwc&hl=en&sa=X&ved=0ahUKEwiB2uDvqIHXAhXCOBoKHdyODXYQ6AEIKDAA#v=onepage&q=%22william%20farr%22%20%22wrecked%20on%20his%20voyage%22&f=false

5. www.health.harvard.edu/newsletter_article/marriage-and-mens-health (article based on www.ncbi.nlm.nih.gov/pubmed/11822923)

6. www.newscientist.com/article/dn3942-masturbating-may-protect-against-prostate-cancer/

7. www.independent.co.uk/life-style/health-and-families/health-news/children-makes-you-live-longer-a7626921.html

8. https://news.byu.edu/news/stayin%E2%80%99-alive-that%E2%80%99s-what-friends-are

9. https://www.psychologytoday.com/blog/wired-success/
    201408/is-there-limit-the-friendships-we-can-maintain

10. See www.theguardian.com/science/2014/feb/16/loneliness-twice-as-
    unhealthy-as-obesity-older-people and www.forbes.com/sites/
    quora/2017/01/18/loneliness-might-be-a-bigger-health-risk-than-
    smoking-or-obesity/#691fb7525d13

11. See http://jamanetwork.com/journals/jamainternalmedicine/
    fullarticle/2521827, www.health.harvard.edu/mind-and-mood/attending-
    religious-services-linked-to-longer-lives-study-shows and http://edition.
    cnn.com/2016/05/16/health/religion-lifespan-health/index.html

12. http://www.telegraph.co.uk/lifestyle/wellbeing/mood-mind/11589864/
    Dont-relax-stress-can-be-good-for-you.html

13. www.ncbi.nlm.nih.gov/pmc/articles/PMC3374921/

14. Saul Bellow, *The Actual* (New York and Harmondsworth: Penguin
    Classics, 1997).

15. https://hbr.org/2016/10/youre-likely-to-live-longer-if-you-retire-after-65

16. www.cambridge.org/core/journals/ageing-and-society/article/does-early-
    retirement-lead-to-longer-life/DBA83CC3D848620FA8EAA
    CEBE9CDE53E

17. http://citeseerx.ist.psu.edu/viewdoc/download?doi=10.1.1.484.1149&rep=
    rep1&type=pdf

18. www3.imperial.ac.uk/newsandeventspggrp/imperialcollege/newssummary/
    news_24-4-2017-17-42-52

19. http://news.bbc.co.uk/1/hi/677048.stm

20. http://news.bbc.co.uk/1/hi/sci/tech/2044646.stm

CHAPTER 11

1. Translated by Stefano Rossoni

2. www.sciencealert.com/scientists-are-investigating-why-people-in-this-
    tiny-italian-town-keep-living-to-100

3. www.telegraph.co.uk/news/2016/09/05/want-to-live-to-be-100-these-
    italian-villagers-may-hold-the-secr/

4. www.independent.co.uk/life-style/health-and-families/health-news/
    scientists-key-to-longevity-italy-acciaroli-centenarian-mediterranean-
    diet-a7230956.html

5. www.bbc.co.uk/news/magazine-30351406

6. www1.cbn.com/cbnnews/healthscience/2015/February/Secrets-to-Longevity-Revealed-in-Denominations-Lifestyle

7. www.alongerhealthylife.com/longevity-village/okinawa-japan-longevity-hotspot/

8. www.telegraph.co.uk/news/health/news/6718612/Village-shows-good-life-holds-secret-to-long-life.html

9. www.thetimes.co.uk/article/air-pollution-on-busy-roads-as-bad-as-passive-smoking-10-a-day-60q2pwdg0

10. www.ilntoday.com/2013/03/few-countries-have-adequate-road-safety-laws/ and www.mshblegal.com/PI-Law-Blogs/Personal-injury-law/few-countries-have-adequate-road-safety-laws.html

11. www.theguardian.com/world/2011/sep/05/september-11-road-deaths

12. www.dailymail.co.uk/femail/article-3172125/Women-underestimate-risk-casual-sex-holiday-leaving-risk-catching-STIs-alcohol-blame.html (from Berdychevsky, L. and Gibson, H.J. (2015) 'Sex and risk in young women's tourist experiences: Context, likelihood, and consequences.' *Tourism Management*, 51: 78–90).

13. https://en.wikipedia.org/wiki/Number_of_terrorist_incidents_by_country

14. www.independent.co.uk/money/pensions/most-britons-prefer-to-retire-abroad-2052834.html and www.express.co.uk/finance/personalfinance/195408/Avoid-perils-of-retiring-abroad

CHAPTER 12

1. www.medicaldaily.com/life-expectancy-injury-high-income-countries-372832 and www.cbsnews.com/news/report-us-life-expectancy-lowest-among-wealthy-nations-due-to-disease-violence/

2. www.cass.city.ac.uk/faculty-and-research/research/cass-knowledge/2016/may/investigating-the-widening-gap-in-life-expectancy-between-richest-and-poorest

3. https://80000hours.org/articles/money-and-happiness/ (download the original article from www.nber.org/papers/w14969)

4. www.dailymail.co.uk/news/article-2054763/Once-million-dollars-hamburger-Bill-Gates-says-billionaire-overrated.html and www.

businessinsider.com/bill-gates-thinks-everyone-only-really-needs-1-million-2011-10?IR=T

5. www.echo-news.co.uk/news/national/13333705.display/

6. Stacey, S. (2013) 'Health Notes: Karren Brady on life after a stroke, relief for kids from chicken pox and relieving facial tension', *Mail on Sunday*, 5 May. At www.dailymail.co.uk/home/you/article-2317799/Health-Notes-Karren-Brady-life-stroke-relief-kids-chicken-pox-relieving-facial-tension.html. See also www.independent.co.uk/sport/football/news-and-comment/karren-brady-grounds-for-optimism-6577523.html

7. www.national-lottery.co.uk/life-changing/winner-millionaire-map

8. https://www.thetimes.co.uk/article/rich-buy-time-as-lifespan-divide-widens-8txb7w08mqi

CHAPTER 14

1. www.dailymail.co.uk/health/article-3185544/The-spicy-food-alive-People-eat-fiery-items-day-reduce-chance-early-death-cancer-heart-disease.html

2. www.theguardian.com/science/neurophilosophy/2014/oct/01/your-nose-knows-death-is-imminent and www.smh.com.au/lifestyle/life/sense-of-smell-may-predict-longevity-university-study-finds-20141002-10pmfd.html

3. http://dca.au.dk/en/current-news/news/show/artikel/ost-er-forbloeffende-sund/ and www.telegraph.co.uk/food-and-drink/news/eat-cheddar-live-longer-5-surprising-health-benefits-cheese/

4. www.telegraph.co.uk/news/health/news/9749949/The-secret-to-why-the-French-live-longer-Roquefort-cheese.html

5. www.jstor.org/stable/41062245?seq=1#page_scan_tab_contents

6. www.nature.com/nature/journal/v333/n6170/abs/333213b0.html?foxtrotcallback=true and see also www.bbc.co.uk/news/magazine-23988352

7. www.theguardian.com/theguardian/2001/feb/05/guardianleaders

8. www.theguardian.com/lifeandstyle/2015/feb/23/saunas-help-you-live-longer-study-finds and www.cbsnews.com/news/spend-time-in-the-sauna-live-longer/

9. http://edition.cnn.com/2016/04/22/health/living-near-nature-linked-to-longer-lives/index.html

10. See www.sciencedirect.com/science/article/pii/S0277953616303689 and www.theguardian.com/books/2016/aug/08/book-up-for-a-longer-life-readers-die-later-study-finds

INDEX